Don't Cross Your Eyes . . .
They'll Get Stuck That Way!

Don't Cross Your Eyes . . .
They'll Get Stuck That Way!

AND 75 OTHER HEALTH MYTHS DEBUNKED

DR. AARON E. CARROLL AND
DR. RACHEL C. VREEMAN

ST. MARTIN'S GRIFFIN ♠ NEW YORK

www.stmartins.com

ISBN 978-0-312-68187-6

First Edition: July 2011

10   9   8   7   6   5   4   3   2   1

Contents

Don't Cross Your Eyes . . .
They'll Get Stuck That Way!

Introduction

Don't cross your eyes . . . they'll get stuck that way!" Did your mother scold you every time you made a crazy face at your brother? In our houses, it was even worse if she caught you sitting too close to the television or she had just caught you reading in the dark. We bet that you still occasionally wonder whether you would need your glasses if you had listened to her.

Your mother had some strong ideas about what would keep you healthy. Use soap! Stay away from that sick person! Don't shake hands! Don't touch the toilet! Her rules for taking care of your body went on and on. Without even realizing it, many of us follow all kinds of rules for keeping our bodies healthy. We worry about how public bathrooms and airplanes might make us sick. We try to stay away from eggs and carbonated drinks. We drink warm milk when we cannot sleep. We tell our own children not to sit too close to the television. We even secretly think that handling a toad might give us warts.

Every day, one hears or reads more ideas about how to care for our bodies. We use hydrogen peroxide to clean out our wounds and vitamin E to heal them faster. We eat oysters to get in the mood. We stretch before running to prevent an injury. Have you ever sniffled or coughed in the wrong company? Vitamin C, echinacea, zinc, and neti pots will immediately be foisted upon you as surefire cures for your cold. As we hear more and more information about our bodies, the list of things to be worried about only grows. You better not eat eggs or hot peppers or sugar or chocolate or fish. Caffeine will stunt your growth. Hair dye will hurt your unborn baby. Cell phones and deodorant might give you cancer. Even worse, the list of things you are supposed to avoid seems to change every day.

Sometimes, though, we worry about the wrong things. We worry about wet hair and accidentally touching a toilet when we should be much more worried about smoking or not exercising regularly. But it is easy to worry about the wrong things when we hear them all the time. Your grandmother, your favorite magazine, and even your doctor all may have told you that eggs will give you high cholesterol or that hot peppers will give you an ulcer. If your snot turns green, everyone will want you to run to the doctor for an antibiotic.

We hope this book provides an antidote to many of your worries. *Don't Cross Your Eyes* outlines why many of the things you heard from your grandmother or your favorite magazine or even your doctor are actually medical myths.

This book is meant to get you to ask questions. What will really make me sick? How does my body really work? What things actually work to keep my body healthy? We don't want to get you in trouble with your mother, but we do want to get you thinking about the truth behind all those crazy things you hear about your body and health. We want you to ask "why?"

Many of the things you hear about your body are just not true. They are myths. Some of the ideas are simply unproven, while others have been studied scientifically and proven false. We think that it is silly to waste time, energy, and money worrying about things that will not hurt you. It is just as silly to follow advice that is not going to help you.

As physicians, we want you to be healthy, and we certainly do not want you to get sick. But because we are also researchers, we want you to know the truth about your body. We want our advice to be based on science. If there is good science telling us what will or will not make your body healthy, we think that you should pay attention to it. In our first book, *Don't Swallow Your Gum! Myths, Half-Truths, and Outright Lies About Your Body and Health*, we discussed dozens of myths about how your body works. In this book, we are going to examine many more of them. We are not just going to be "experts" telling you what will or will not work to keep you healthy. We are going to explore the science behind various ideas about your health, and we will let the science tell you what you can stop worrying about.

Even though we are doctors (and true geeks) who get excited about research studies and scientific experiments, we know that not everyone feels that way. (Aaron just shed a sad geek tear thinking about people who don't like science.) Nonetheless, this book—about all the crazy things your mother said about your body—is secretly a science book. We researched each of the ideas in depth, combing the medical and scientific literature for any studies that have been done to tell us the truth about these medical beliefs. Then we try to describe the research in a way that allows you to understand what it says.

Remember, we want you to ask "why?" We don't want you to believe something is a myth just because *we* said so. We want you to understand *why* we said so. That is why we will talk about the research behind each belief and whether good studies give us an answer. Most of the beliefs we examine in this list from A to Z end up being completely false. They are myths or outright lies! Others have some element of the truth. Just a few actually turn out to be true. Whatever the case, we want you to know whether the science comes out in favor or against the belief, and just how convincing the case may be. In the back of the book, you can find a big list of the references for what we say about each myth. We are always scouring the databases for new studies that add more information, and if new studies come out that prove an idea is or is not true, we are happy to change our minds based on that research.

Before you start reading, we offer two words of caution. First of all, some readers of *Don't Swallow Your Gum!* told us that the book turned them into the know-it-all at the dinner table or at the party. We love being right, but we also know that people can get annoyed when you are always Ms. or Mr. Smarty-pants. Use discretion. Second, it is always a good idea to show respect for your mother. Even if she is wrong.

Happy myth-busting!

Acupuncture

You know what'll really get rid of that cold? . . . Acupuncture

No one likes having a cold. Whether you hate the cough and sore throat the most, or whether it is the sniffling and congestion that wears you out, you want that cold to be finished as soon as possible. Here in the United States, you may be more likely to try vitamin C or echinacea, but in other parts of the world, such as in Japan and China, acupuncture is a more common alternative therapy for cold relief.

In careful studies, acupuncture has been shown to work for a number of medical problems. It can be an effective way to treat the nausea that many people feel after they have surgery and anesthesia. It can cut down on the vomiting that cancer patients experience when they are getting chemotherapy. It can help with some kinds of pain, including childbirth, pain from shoulder or neck injuries, and chronic back pain. But acupuncture does not work for every problem. In studies where acupuncture was used to treat cocaine addiction, depression, insomnia, or irritable bowel syndrome, it did not help patients.

Few cold remedies actually work, so it is not surprising people would want to give acupuncture a whirl. Unfortunately, there is very little evidence that acupuncture works to prevent or treat colds. In the medical literature, most of the studies using acupuncture in this way come from Japan. Two of them examined whether acupuncture could prevent people from catching colds. Both of these "studies" showed that acupuncture was useful for preventing colds, but we put the word "studies" in quotation marks for a good reason: they were only case reports of people who had used acupuncture frequently and seemed to have fewer colds. In fact, the two reports only looked at three people. The experiences of three people are not enough to decide whether a cold prevention method works and should not be counted as actual research.

A final study from Japan looked at whether the students and staff in five Japanese acupuncture schools had any fewer colds or any fewer cold symptoms if they received acupuncture. This study included more people (326). Although those receiving acupuncture did report fewer cold symptoms in an overall questionnaire, there was no difference in how many days the participants were reporting cold symptoms in daily diary records.

There were several other problems with this study. First, the most accurate measure of whether the people in the study were having cold symptoms did not show any improvement with acupuncture. The participants only thought there was a difference when they were asked about the overall picture. This might be explained in part by another problem with the methodology: there was no fake acupuncture, or placebo, used for the group that did not get acupuncture for cold symptoms. The people who had acupuncture knew that they had had acupuncture, and so it is possible that they remembered differently because they thought the acupuncture had made things better. The study was also flawed because there were significant differences in the groups being studied even before the study began.

There is no good evidence to suggest that acupuncture will stop you from catching a cold or that it will make your cold symptoms any better. While acupuncture could be studied more carefully for coughs and colds, as it has been for other health problems, there is no convincing reason to believe (yet) that acupuncture is just the thing for your cold.

ADHD

ADHD medication will stunt your child's growth

More than four million children in the United States have been diagnosed with Attention Deficit/Hyperactivity Disorder (ADHD). For children with ADHD, particular types of stimulant medications have been proven to be effective therapies in managing their symptoms. While many parents and doctors appreciate how these medicines help children overcome the hyperactivity, distractibility, or inattention that come with ADHD, they worry about how the medicines for ADHD might also be harmful. In particular, many parents and doctors alike have heard that ADHD medicines stunt children's growth. Parents rightfully wonder whether the benefits outweigh the risks.

Many studies have investigated the question of whether ADHD medicines stunt children's growth. Several studies have found statistically significant changes in the height and weight of children treated for ADHD; children who are taking ADHD medicines do appear to have slower increases in height and weight as they age. However, the medicine's effect on growth wanes over time. In a review examining twenty studies of children's growth while taking ADHD medicines, it was learned that there were some delays in the children's growth in terms of height and weight gain, but these effects became less or went away over time. In other words, the medicines seemed to slow down the children's growth at first, but then that effect diminished. Several studies also suggested that the dosage is what has the greater effect on the child's growth. It is important to note that the differences in the children's growth compared to children not on medicines for ADHD were very small, and some of the studies suggested that the children went on to have normal adult height and weight. The summary of all these studies is that there seems to be some impact from ADHD medicine on children's growth, but the effect is less over time and may not have any impact on how tall they are as adults.

There are also some studies that suggest that the medicines are not the real culprit for the children's growth, and that the real issue may be the fact that they have ADHD. In some studies, ADHD itself is associated with alterations in how children grow, even among children who have never received medication for their ADHD. Most of the studies from which scientists try to answer this question were not really intended to see whether ADHD alone affects children's growth, and so more research is needed in order to provide a definitive answer.

If you are considering ADHD treatment for your child, you should be aware that there is some potential for a temporary growth delay, especially when they first start therapy. However, you should also know that most of these growth delays go away over time and the child usually catches up in terms of their growth. It is also important to weigh any of these risks against the very real problems that children with ADHD have when they are not treated with medication. These problems include not only difficulties in school, but also a higher chance of having issues such as depression, anxiety, and difficulty relating to their peers.

Air

The air you breathe will make you sick . . . if you're near a sniffler and sneezer

Your co-worker is coughing and sneezing in the cubicle just down the way. The sniffling and throat-clearing make it difficult to concentrate. You are worried about getting sick yourself, but the etiquette of asking someone to go home or to stay in bed is tricky to navigate. Some of your colleagues are ready to march the snot-nosed sicko out the door, but you wonder just how much of a problem it really is to breathe the same air. You use your hand sanitizer, try to avoid being within sneezing range of their red nose, and you definitely are not shaking hands—but are you still at risk of catching their cold?

Unfortunately, the answer to this one is "maybe." Sometimes, breathing the same air as a sick person will make you sick. The viruses that most often cause colds in humans are called rhinoviruses. For a long time, it looked like the main way that rhinoviruses were passed from one human being to another was through direct contact. The rhinoviruses most often passed from one person to another by directly touching things that had been contaminated by coughing and sneezing. This is why handwashing is so important. Your hands typically touch contaminated objects, and when you put your hands in your mouth or nose, the virus creeps in to infect you. A sick person's hands are also a big culprit of passing on cold viruses. Coughing and sneezing into your hands covers them with tiny (or, sometimes, not so tiny) droplets of mucus that contain the cold virus. When you touch things with your contaminated hands, you leave behind infectious mucus that can get other people sick. Washing hands and avoiding contact with a sick person's contaminated hands or the things their hands may have touched are still the most important ways to avoid catching another person's cold.

If cold viruses were only passed from person to person by direct contact, then you would not have to worry much about breathing the same air. You could just wash your hands and keep a little distance, and you would be fine. However, more recent studies have shown that some cold viruses are aerosolized. This means that the virus is sent into the air in small droplets of fluid that come spewing out of your mouth or nose when you cough or sneeze. With this kind of transmission, you're most at risk if you are very close to that coughing or sneezing person. With some bad luck, you might get these virus-containing droplets of fluid into your nose or mouth.

But what about someone who is not within spitting range? Are you in danger just by breathing in the same air? This is where newer studies give us especially bad news. There is evidence that some viruses get aerosolized into the air in a way that allows them to circulate through buildings, and even to infect people who are not particularly close by. Many of the buildings in which we spend our time are relatively well sealed. They have central heating, ventilation, and air-conditioning, and the indoor air circulates around the building for some time before it is exchanged for the air outside. In these conditions, it appears that some viruses get circulated in the indoor air and cause infections in other people in the building.

It is much more likely that you will be infected by someone near you or by the mucus that someone leaves on your hands or on your phone, but there is a chance that you might get sick from someone on another floor too. Good ventilation systems can do a lot to prevent the spread of sickness through the air. If the system frequently exchanges indoor air for outdoor air, it can prevent most of these infections that spread through the air.

These studies are looking at colds or upper respiratory infections caused by viruses, and not at other types of sicknesses. Many other forms of illness, such as diarrhea or strep throat or skin infections, are not spread through the air. These illnesses are usually spread by direct contact, and so the air around people with these sicknesses is not going to make you sick. And other illnesses are not contagious at all and cannot be passed from one person to another. For example, you cannot get heart failure, diabetes, or leukemia from another person.

Those of us who work in hospitals and breathe in "sick air" all the time can easily avoid getting sick ourselves. There's no trick to it. We follow the same recommendations we give you in this book and in *Don't Swallow Your Gum!*: wash your hands frequently, get a flu shot, and if you have to be around someone who has a cold or viral respiratory infection, wear a mask or try to give them more personal space.

Airborne

Airborne is a popular supplement among schoolteachers, who claim that it prevents them from picking up the germs spread around their classrooms full of sick children. The Airborne package even tells the story of how it was created by a schoolteacher who was frustrated with just that problem—getting sick all the time during cold and flu season. Rachel flies a lot, and friends and family who want to be helpful are always suggesting that she should take Airborne before she gets on one of her long plane rides. If Airborne works for teachers and travelers, it should work for you, right? The problem is, there is no evidence that it works.

It may surprise you to hear that Airborne has not been studied scientifically. Since Airborne is a herbal supplement, it is not regulated by the U.S. Food and Drug Administration (FDA), and its makers are not required to tell us exactly what is in it or whether it is proven to work. We know that Airborne contains a mixture of vitamins, minerals, and herbs, including large amounts of vitamin C and vitamin A, as well as some zinc. In the medical literature, there are no studies of Airborne itself. We can assure you that if someone had done a good scientific study and proved that this worked, it would be published prominently. Of course, some of the components of Airborne have been studied rigorously. As you will see if you skip to some of the later chapters, studies show over and over again that vitamin C, echinacea, and zinc do not prevent or cure colds. If the individual components of Airborne do not work to prevent colds, it seems unlikely that Airborne itself will work.

If you are a fan of Airborne, you may be shocked by our claim that Airborne has not been studied. After all, the package used to talk about the "double-blind, placebo-controlled clinical trial of 120 patients" that showed Airborne worked great in helping patients in the early stages of getting a cold. The makers of Airborne had to remove that claim because, as it turns out, the "study" was conducted unscientifically. In fact, as uncovered by an investigative report by ABC News, the scientific team at GNG Pharmaceutical Services were, in fact, two men working in a garage. The scientific studies that we use for evidence in this book are done in clinics and controlled laboratories by scientists and doctors. They are not done by two men in a garage. The makers of Airborne agreed to pay more than $24 million to settle a class-action lawsuit in regard to their false advertising about this garage "study" and the lack of evidence for their product.

As the Federal Trade Commission summarizes, the makers of Airborne cannot make any legitimate claims about the effectiveness of their products: "There is no competent and reliable scientific evidence to support the claims made by the defendants that Airborne tablets can prevent or reduce the risk of colds, sickness, or infection; protect against or help fight germs; reduce the severity or duration of a cold; and protect against colds, sickness, or infection in crowded places such as airplanes, offices, or schools."

The FTC complaint also states that the individual defendants in the case, company founders Victoria Knight-McDowell and Thomas John McDowell, made false claims that Airborne products are clinically proven to treat colds.

We kind of like the idea of a plucky schoolteacher figuring out a way to treat colds effectively. What we detest is the idea that someone could make a fortune lying to people about whether something works. The Federal Trade Commission reports that lying is exactly what the makers of Airborne did, and they had to pay millions in order to settle the lawsuit caused by those lies.

The other thing we don't like is that products like Airborne are not without risk. It is bad enough if something doesn't work, but much worse if it could also make you sick. Since Airborne is not proven to work, we cannot be sure how much risk of a harmful side effect you might have from taking it. In these instances, vulnerable populations like pregnant women and children need to be especially careful because we just don't know what the impact of this product might be.

Airborne is not proven to work. Existing studies of the components of Airborne suggest that it is unlikely to work even if it was rigorously studied. And the makers of Airborne have consistently lied about its effectiveness. All of these things add up to a product that does not deserve to be trusted (or foisted upon unsuspecting airplane seatmates).

Airplanes

Airplane travel will make you sick

Rachel spends half of the year doing research and caring for children with HIV in Kenya. Going back and forth to Africa several times a year means a lot of time on airplanes (and a lot of frequent flier miles). Does it also mean that Rachel has a lot of extra colds? Rachel's family is convinced that she is always coming off airplane flights with some sort of sickness. If Airborne is not going to protect her on the plane, is she doomed to exposure to one germ after another?

Many people are convinced that airplanes are guaranteed incubators for coughs and colds. Vice President Joe Biden once warned family members that they should avoid airplanes during the time of the swine flu epidemic because a single sneeze in the confined space of a plane could go "all the way through the aircraft." The makers of Airborne particularly recommend taking their herbal supplement before you fly on a plane in order to prevent colds. One has to wonder just how significant the health risks are when you fly.

It is easy to imagine how airplanes could be incubators for illness. Airplanes are confined spaces, and they have limited ventilation. People worry that the airplane ventilation systems may recirculate stale cabin air. Plus, if you have a long flight, you may be close to a sick person for a relatively long time.

Studies have found some evidence that traveling on a plane can lead to infections among other air travelers. Studies looking at the transmission of pandemic A/H1N1 influenza (swine flu) in 2009 did show an increased chance of getting swine flu if you were in close proximity to a passenger on an airplane who was already infected. For swine flu, the risk was only increased for those people within two rows of the sick passengers. There are also case reports of diseases such as tuberculosis, measles, and other types of influenza being transmitted from one passenger on a plane to another. We have to admit that air travel can be a risk. (This is also a good reminder to get vaccinated against whatever infections you can since you never know what the person next to you on a plane might have.)

Before you cancel your next flight, though, you should look at the big picture. Air travel is not nearly as risky as it may sound. Bugs and viruses are actually spread during flight very rarely. You put yourself at risk for getting an infection whenever you go out in public. Studies show that you have no more risk of getting sick after being on an airplane than you do if you spend the same amount of time on trains, buses, or in buildings like offices or malls. Airplanes are not the worst culprits. In fact, one study found lower levels of bacteria and fungi in airplanes than in buses, malls, or even in the outside air! Studies that look at cultures from airplanes show very low levels of growing bacteria or viruses. Airplanes have a number of factors in their favor that help to keep them much healthier than you might imagine.

First of all, the air in the cabin of an airplane is really quite clean. The cabin air originally comes from the air outside the plane, which is at very high altitude. High altitude air starts off with very few bacteria and viruses in it. Then, the air is compressed and heated before it gets sent into the cabin, a process that should also kill remaining bacteria or viruses. So the air that comes into the airplane for you to breathe is actually very clean. Of course, the next step is for that clean air to start recirculating in a cabin that may include sick people. Some risk enters the picture with the recirculation, but the risk is really very low. Within an airplane's recirculation system, the air is filtered through a system of high efficiency particulate air (HEPA)–type filters. These filters are very good at removing bacteria and even viruses from the air; they are better than the filters in most buildings, and are the same kinds of filters used to clean the air in hospital wards or operating rooms. Therefore, both the air coming into the plane from outside and the recirculated air once inside are very clean overall.

To make the ride in the plane even safer, the air in the cabin is exchanged very frequently, typically twenty times in an hour. This is much better than most office buildings, where air is exchanged twelve times in an hour, or most houses, where air is exchanged five times in an hour. The air circulation system also tries to avoid sending the air all around the plane. Instead, the air that leaves from a particular row, after being cleaned, comes back to that particular row. The air exchange moves from the top to the bottom of the plane, rather than from the front to the back. If any germs manage to get into the air, they stay pretty close to the infected person, instead of traveling all through the plane. The current airplane recirculation systems seem to work pretty well. In fact, in a study of airplane air circulation, there was no difference in how many respiratory symptoms passengers developed if they were on a plane that recirculated air compared to a plane that had no recirculation and only used new air from outside.

But perhaps you've felt ill in other ways after you've flown. While the plane may not be a dangerous incubator for colds, there are some other ways in which flying might affect you. While it's quite clean, the air on the plane is also very dry. This actually helps prevent infections because bacteria and viruses like to live in tiny water droplets in more humid air, but the dry air might make your nose and throat dry too. Having a dry nose and throat could lead to bothersome irritation of your sinuses and respiratory system. Some researchers speculate that dry, irritated mucus membranes might make it easier for you to get infected with a cold later on, but this has not been proven.

Traveling on long flights in an airplane can also put you at risk for developing a blood clot in your leg (called a deep vein thrombosis or DVT). DVT can result from long periods of time where you have to sit still or are not able to move as much, such as being in bed after surgery or sitting still on a long airplane ride. Flexing your legs frequently and walking around when you can on a long plane ride are smart ways to try to prevent developing DVT.

There have also been cases where people on a particular flight later developed diarrhea and vomiting after one passenger had been very sick in the airplane bathroom. Unfortunately, contamination of the bathroom and subsequent poor hand-washing by others caused this infection to spread. You can imagine how gross that bathroom must have been! Contaminated bathrooms anywhere can cause infections to spread, so wash your hands and try not to touch obviously dirty stuff.

So, as it turns out, airplanes are not so icky after all. People worry about the quality of air in airplanes and about how likely they are to get sick from their time on the plane, but the studies of airplane ventilation systems and of who gets sick after air travel both suggest that we are a lot more worried than we need to be. Although it is possible to have infections pass among passengers on airplanes, there are many precautions in place that help make this a low risk. The heating of almost sterile outside air, the filtration systems, the low humidity, and the patterns of airflow in the plane all minimize the chance of spreading infections among passengers. Even for frequent fliers, the risk of being on a plane does not seem to be any greater than the risk of being on a train or bus or even the risk from going to the office.

Aloe Vera

Aloe vera will heal a burn—TRUE

Aaron was *sure* this one would turn out to be a myth. So many of the home remedies or cures we hear about do not work when they are tested scientifically. He thought aloe vera would turn out to be another of those good-sounding but not-working remedies. But after carefully reviewing the medical literature, it does appear to be true, that aloe vera is good for burns.

There have been a number of excellent studies that have looked at how aloe vera works on burns. In one of these, published in *Surgery Today* in 2009, thirty patients with two second degree burns on their bodies had one burn treated with aloe vera and the other treated with silver sulfadiazine (a long accepted cream for burns). The rate of developing new skin cells and the time to complete healing were about three days faster for those burns treated with aloe vera. Aloe vera worked!

This confirmed the findings from earlier studies, like one published in the *Journal of the Medical Association of Thailand*. Patients with significant burns called partial thickness burns were treated with aloe vera or standard Vaseline gauze. Those who used the aloe vera saw their wounds heal six days faster.

In fact, there have been enough studies of burn-healing with aloe vera that a systematic review and meta-analysis has been published. In these types of studies, researchers compile all the studies that have been done to evaluate whether something does or does not work, and draw a conclusion from the combined data. By looking at the total evidence, the researchers concluded that aloe vera led to burns healing almost nine days faster on average.

Additionally, aloe vera doesn't seem to have any significant side effects. Sure, it's not the treatment of choice for very severe burns, or those requiring a hospitalization, but for most first and second degree burns it seems to work really well. Go ahead and use it!

Antibiotics

Antibiotics kill the germs that cause colds and the flu

A ntibiotics kill bacteria or stop them from growing so that our bodies can be cleared of bacterial infections. They are, without a doubt, one of the best advances of modern medicine. Bacteria can cause infections in many different places in our bodies, and some of these infections can be serious. Antibiotics (you can think of the name as meaning "anti-bacteria") help our bodies to fight off bacterial infections that the body might not be able to handle by itself. Different antibiotics work for different types of bacteria. When you are sick with an infection from a bacterium, your doctor has to think about what kinds of bacteria usually cause that kind of infection and then pick an antibiotic that should work to kill those particular bacteria. So, antibiotics CAN kill a lot of germs, if you think of germs as bacteria.

As great as antibiotics are for killing bacteria, antibiotics cannot kill viruses. Viruses and bacteria are not the same. While both are germs that can make us sick, they look and act in very different ways. Viruses are teeny-tiny little, special, small machines that can enter into the cells in your body and use your body's own equipment to make you sick. You could imagine a virus like a special computer that has been programmed to take over the master controls of a big ship just by being hooked up to the control panel. In contrast, a bacterium would be more like an evil person who snuck inside the ship's control room and is making decisions about what to sabotage and how to maneuver the ship. Bacteria are full-fledged organisms in a way that viruses are not; a virus is more like a nefariously programmed computer, whereas bacteria are more like evil villains. As you might imagine, the methods you would use to stop or kill that evil person are different from the methods you would use to deal with the computer. Antibiotics cannot kill the "computer" even if they work great against the "villain."

Antibiotics cannot kill viruses. Antibiotics only kill infections caused by bacteria, fungi, and some parasites. Because antibiotics work for some infections (those caused by bacteria) and not for other infections (those cause by viruses), it is important to know what is causing your infection. Colds and the flu are caused by viruses, not by bacteria. Viruses also cause most coughs and sore throats.

Since colds and the flu are caused by viruses, antibiotics do not treat them. If you have a cold or the flu, an antibiotic will not help you feel any better. It will not make you better faster. It will not prevent you from spreading the cold or flu to anyone else. It will not kill your germs.

If you are infected with a virus, the only thing that an antibiotic might do is make you feel worse. Why is that? The antibiotic is not going to do a thing to help with your cough or cold symptoms, but it might cause some unpleasant side effects, such as diarrhea or rashes. It could also kill off the good bacteria that normally live inside your digestive tract or other parts of your body, leaving you with a yeast infection or an overgrowth of bad bacteria in the place of your body's usual good bacteria.

When we use antibiotics when they are not needed, bacteria that are in your body but not causing disease can learn to be resistant to them. Bacteria that have not been killed off by an antibiotic may learn how to survive against it. If you think of the evil person trying to take control of your ship, it would be like that person saw your fighting style once, but you did not kill him, and so now he knows how to defend himself against you in the future. Using antibiotics when they are not needed or using them improperly, by not taking enough of them, or not taking them for as long as you are supposed to, allows resistant bacteria to develop. When you get infected by one of these resistant bacteria, it can cause serious problems because our usual antibiotics do not work.

So the bottom line here is that it really is important to use antibiotics properly. If your doctor says that you do not need an antibiotic, you shouldn't demand one. You should not be taking an antibiotic for a viral infection like a cold or for most sore throats or coughs. If the doctor is not sure whether your infection is caused by a bacterium or a virus, this is something you can talk about together in order to decide on a plan.

Additionally, you should never take antibiotics that are prescribed for someone else. As we mentioned, antibiotics are not all the same. They work in very particular ways for particular bugs. An antibiotic prescribed for someone else might not work for your infection, even if your infection is caused by bacteria. It might also make your bacteria mutate into resistant bacteria. And it might make it difficult for your doctor to know what is infecting you.

Taking antibiotics properly also means taking an antibiotic for the entire prescribed period. Even if you or your child feels much better, you should take the antibiotic for the entire time that the doctor suggests. Do your very best not to skip any doses of the medicine. When you skip doses, the bacteria have a chance to grow and become resistant when less of the drug is present in your body.

Antibiotics are wonderful medicines. People used to die from simple infections that we can easily treat today. We should not expect antibiotics to work for things that they are not designed to kill, and we should not use antibiotics in ways that will ruin their usefulness by causing resistance. If you have a cold or the flu, antibiotics will not work! Never, ever, ever! Taking an antibiotic for a virus might even do more harm than good.

Once an individual has started a course of antibiotics, he is no longer contagious

When one child in the playgroup is sick with something, the other parents often go into hyperalert mode. They want to make sure their children stay far away from a contagious child or anything that he or she might touch. Once that child is on an antibiotic, though, the vigilance relaxes. Once the antibiotic starts, schools and day cares and colleagues relax. Just the words "I'm on an antibiotic" are enough to make most of the hypochondriacs around you relax.

Being contagious means that you are able to spread your disease to other people. Unfortunately for people trying hard to avoid getting sick, it is not always simple to determine when someone is contagious and when they are not. Antibiotics might help, but they often don't.

First of all, for viral infections, especially the viruses that cause most of our colds and the flu, antibiotics will never, ever make you less contagious. Antibiotics only work against bacteria; they do not work against viruses. If a person is sick with a virus, an antibiotic will do nothing to make them less contagious. Another problem is that the time period when you are contagious varies according to what type of sickness you have. An ill person can be contagious before they show any symptoms. When you are infected with a virus, you typically shed or spread the virus for at least a day or two before you have any idea you're sick. The virus is in anything coming out of your mouth or nose during this time, even before you are coughing and sneezing. Then, when your nose first starts running or you have any other symptoms, you shed even more of the virus. Even as you start feeling better, you might still be contagious and spreading the virus eight or ten days after your sickness starts.

This type of spread is true for both the viruses that cause coughs and colds, as well as viruses that cause infections like herpes. The virus can spread before you have any signs of the infection. Infections such as chickenpox, fifth disease, and some forms of meningitis may all be contagious before you have any symptoms. On the other hand, other viral infections, such as the main virus that causes pinkeye, do not spread before the person actually develops symptoms.

Don't vow to stay in your house and shun other people forever! Even though antibiotics are not going to protect you from their coughs, colds, and crud, it is also important to realize that many illnesses are not contagious at all—even some very serious infections. Ear infections, sinus infections, and urinary tract infections happen as a result of a passageway or tube being blocked by an overgrowth of bacteria. These types of infections are usually not contagious. You need antibiotics to kill off the bacteria growing in your ear or in your bladder for you to feel better, but you are not going to pass this infection to someone else if you do not have an antibiotic. Other serious infections, such as infections of your bloodstream or pneumonias, are not very contagious to other people. Most often, these infections come about because of something else that was going on in your body first, and so healthy people around you are unlikely to get infected by the same thing. For other infections, like most sexually transmitted diseases, you will not get infected unless you have sexual contact with the person infected or have some other very close contact with them.

Clearly, though, there are bacterial infections that can spread from one person to another. In these cases, you do want the sick person to be on an antibiotic so that they do not infect you. One of the bacteria that causes meningitis, *Neisseria meningitidis*, is contagious, and if one person becomes sick with infection from this bug, that sick person needs an antibiotic, plus close family members exposed to that person need to take antibiotics themselves to prevent infection. In the case of *Neisseria,* it is very good news to know that the infected person is on an antibiotic. Strep throat is another example where having the person on antibiotics may or may not help you. Strep throat is caused by a bacterium, *Streptococcus pyogenes*, and it is contagious. This bug rapidly colonizes the family members and close contacts of the person who has the first infection. When one person in the family has strep throat, the risk that someone else in the family will get strep throat is at least 10 percent. Using an antibiotic may help decrease how the bacteria colonize your throat and thus prevent other people from getting infected. The real reason we use antibiotics for strep throat is to prevent other complications to your heart or kidneys that can result without treatment. In contrast to strep throat, another form of the strep bug, *Streptococcus pneumoniae,* which can cause bad pneumonias, is not as contagious as the bug that causes strep throat. While you would certainly need antibiotics to help with one of these strep infections, the antibiotics would not have much of an effect on how contagious you were.

You may have noticed that we said antibiotics "might" make you less contagious, even with contagious bacterial infections like strep throat. The truth is that there are very few scientific studies giving clear data about just how long you remain contagious. Parents are typically told that their child is no longer contagious after they have been on antibiotics for twenty-four hours or sometimes after forty-eight hours. These figures are very roughly based on how fast the antibiotics decrease the load of bacteria within the body. For some conditions, a person might still be contagious with only a small amount of the bacteria around and after they have been on an antibiotic for a while. For other conditions, the person may never have been very contagious or the period of being contagious might have passed even before you started the antibiotic. Some infections are still contagious as long as you have a rash or have a cough, whereas others are not. Often, doctors really do not know just how long you will be contagious. While it is important to take antibiotics for certain medical problems and to take them as directed by your physician, this is not a guaranteed way to know whether someone is contagious.

Whenever you have an infection, you should talk with your doctor about how contagious this infection is, how long it will be contagious, and what, if anything, you need to do to prevent other people from being infected.

Apples

An apple a day keeps the doctor away

Rachel loves apples and has eaten an apple a day for most of her life. She may have become an apple aficionado in her early days because of all of the orchards where she grew up in Grand Rapids, Michigan. Despite this love of apples, Rachel hasn't managed to keep the doctor(s) away. Seriously though—the belief that "an apple a day will keep the doctor away" might not be something to laugh at. Scientists have done a lot of research to determine what is in apples and how they might benefit us. While an apple a day is not going to cure or prevent all of your medical problems, it turns out that apples are a good part of a healthy diet.

Food science examines many potential ways in which apples can help you. In general, there is plenty of evidence to suggest that eating fruits and vegetables is good for you. People who eat diets that are high in fruits and vegetables have less cancer and less heart disease. Scientists generally explain this because fruits and vegetables have certain chemicals, such as phenolics, flavonoids, and carotenoids, all of which are thought to reduce your chances of developing certain chronic diseases. People who eat lots of fruits and vegetables also tend to be slimmer, and that lowers your chances of developing other diseases as well.

What is the evidence for eating an apple a day? Researchers have looked at a lot of epidemiologic studies (studies of large groups of people) to see whether apple eaters might do better than apple scorners. In these studies, eating apples was associated with fewer cases of certain cancers, as well as fewer cases of heart disease, asthma, and diabetes. In a study of 77,000 women and 47,000 men surveyed through the Nurses' Health Study, people who ate one serving a day of apples and pears had fewer instances of lung cancer. In a Finnish study of 10,000 men and women, those who ate the most flavonoids (which were mostly coming from apples and onions) also had the lowest rates of lung cancer. An apple plus a pear plus an onion keeps the doctor away? These are big studies, which are always good, but they do not really test if apples "work" to keep you healthy. It is possible that people who choose to eat apples also choose to do other healthy things that keep them in good shape.

A number of case-control studies have also tried to look at the apple question. In these studies, researchers take people with cancer and people without cancer and ask them about what they have eaten. In a study of patients with and without lung cancer, those who remembered eating the most apples, onions, and white grapefruit had the lowest risk of lung cancer. In a study of patients with and without colorectal cancer, those who ate more than one apple a day (one apple a day was not good enough) had fewer instances of colorectal cancer. These studies suggest that there might be benefit to eating a bunch of apples, but it is also important to remember that the cancer patients' recall of what they ate might be skewed by the fact that they have been diagnosed with cancer. It's easy for people who have cancer to start worrying that they were not healthy enough before their diagnosis; that they didn't eat enough fruits and vegetables, for example, and blame those bad habits for their cancer. This can throw off our understanding of the studies' reports.

There is also some evidence that apples are good for your heart. In the Women's Health Study, which surveyed 40,000 people, eating flavonoids (which are contained in apples) was tied to having fewer "cardiovascular events" even though how many flavonoids you ate did not decrease how many strokes, heart attacks, or deaths from cardiac problems you had. In a study from Finland, women who reported eating fewer apples and onions (combining the apples and onions again!) also had lower rates of type 2 diabetes and more deaths from heart issues, though there was no difference for men. In a study from Iowa, women who ate more apples and drank more wine had lower risks of death from coronary artery disease. (Combining apples and wine sounds much better than combining apples and onions!)

Of course, apples are not the only good-for-you foods out there. Bran, pears, wine, grapefruit, strawberries, and chocolate are also high-flavonoid foods, and eating more of them is also associated with less heart disease and/or lower death rates. Apples might even be good for your lungs if you *also* eat pears. In a study of 1,601 adults in Australia, eating more fruits and vegetables in total was not connected with having or not having asthma. However, the people who ate more apples and pears in specific had lower rates of asthma and wheezing problems. Studies from the Netherlands and Britain also found better pulmonary function among Dutch people who ate more apples and pears, and among British people who ate five apples a week.

There are some scientific reasons why apples might be connected to lower rates of disease. Apples do have lots of chemicals that scientists think are healthy for your body. When researchers analyze apples, they find that apples have lots of good antioxidants, which have names you might not recognize: flavonoid, quercetin, catechin, phloridzin, and chlorogenic. The apple peel has the highest level of these chemicals. Those of us who are not nutritionists may not know what to think of these chemicals, but in the laboratory these chemicals from apples have been shown to be good antioxidants and can even be used to inhibit the growth of some kinds of cancer cells. When food scientists test apple chemicals or apple juice in rats, they can reduce the cholesterol in fat rats, and rats with a disease that is kind of like Alzheimer's do better in running through a maze. (It is important to point out that these studies were, not surprisingly, commissioned by the apple industry.) This evidence all sounds great. Apples contain good things, and they seem to do good things for rats. Are apples really the key to health?

The science lab also offers some evidence that apples are not the perfect cure for human beings. Even though apples have all of these great antioxidant chemicals, your body may not be able to absorb and process them the way it would need for the apple to make a big difference. Some of the chemicals in apples do not seem to be absorbed well by the body (in other words, the chemicals are not very bioavailable). In more than one study of the apple antioxidant called quercetin, they could not find the antioxidant in volunteers' plasma even after they drank 1.1 liters of apple cider or ate a whole apple. Quercetin is mostly found in the apple peel, however, and one study did find this antioxidant in the subjects' plasma after they ate a serving of applesauce plus the apple peel. An antioxidant like quercetin may look great in the laboratory, but if you do not actually absorb it into your bloodstream, it probably will not do you much good. Apples and onions both contain a decent amount of quercetin, but stinky onions might be the better way to get this antioxidant. The amount of quercetin available from apples is only 30 percent of what is available from onions. The other apple all-star chemicals are not absorbed so well either. In a study in rats, the researchers could not find any phloridzin in the rats' plasma after eating apples, even though apples have plenty of this chemical.

The bottom line is that apples are a great fruit; they are healthy to eat and may even have some added benefits for staying well. But you should not think of the apple as a clear-cut way to stay healthy or to improve your health. The studies connecting eating apples with having fewer cancer or heart disease risks are a bit difficult to interpret because the same people choosing to eat more apples are usually also making other healthy choices, such as exercising or not smoking. Plus, people may not remember exactly how much fruit they ate and might inflate the number of apples they report. Ultimately, if you like apples, eat more of them! If you are not an apple fan, do what you can to increase the amount of fruits and vegetables you eat in a day. Other fruits and vegetables and other healthy diet choices might help to keep the doctor away. Onion anyone?

Artificial Sweeteners

Artificial sweeteners will give you cancer

This one will undoubtedly inspire a lot of hate mail. It's one of those myths that has left the realm of science and entered the realm of faith. We take on this chapter knowing that for many of you, no matter what we say, you are going to remain convinced that artificial sweeteners are linked to cancer. However, as we mentioned in the introduction, we do not want you to waste time being needlessly worried about things that are harmless.

Not all artificial sweeteners are the same. Saccharin is one of the oldest. There have been more than fifty studies about the effect of saccharin on rats. About twenty of them involved rats consuming saccharin for at least one and a half years. Nineteen of these studies found no relationship between saccharin and cancer. One study found an increased rate of bladder cancer, but it was in a type of rat that easily gets infected with a bladder parasite that can leave it more susceptible to disease.

Scientists then moved on to see if giving two generations of rats saccharin would do anything. They fed rats, and then their children, lots of saccharin. They found that male rats in the second generation got more bladder cancer. As a result, some countries banned saccharin, and others—like the U.S.—started labeling products with warnings. There was one problem: the link between saccharin and cancer couldn't be found in humans. Later work found that often cancer induced in rats doesn't equal cancer in humans. For instance, if you give rats vitamin C in the same doses as they used for saccharin in the other studies, vitamin C causes bladder cancer in rats too. Yet no one is attempting to ban vitamin C.

Cyclamate is another kind of artificial sweetener that was approved by the FDA for use in the United States in 1950. Almost twenty years later, a landmark study found that cyclamate also increased the rate of bladder cancer in rats. This led to cyclamate being banned in a number of countries. Later, the ban was lifted pretty much everywhere but in the United States. In one of those studies you can't believe they actually did, some scientists fed thirty-seven monkeys either no cyclamate, 100 mg/kg of cyclamate, or 500 mg/kg a cyclamate every day for twenty-four years. Twenty-four years! By the way, 500 mg/kg is like drinking thirty cans of diet soda a day. That's a lot of cyclamate! At the end of the study, they killed the monkeys who had not yet died and autopsied all of them. Three animals that had been given cyclamate had cancers, but they were different types of cancer in different parts of the body, and they were common cancers in monkeys. The conclusion from this long research study was that there was no apparent increased risk of developing cancer—even after consuming that much cyclamate.

Which brings us to aspartame. Approved for use in 1981, it wasn't until 1996 when folks started worrying about aspartame containing carcinogens. In that year, a paper was published that got a lot of attention. This paper discussed the fact that there had been a recent increase in the incidence of brain tumors and questioned whether this could be linked to aspartame. As usually happens with these kinds of things, the media had a field day and people began to panic. But here's the clincher: further investigations of National Cancer Institute statistics showed that the increase in brain tumors began in 1973, eight years before aspartame was introduced. Also, most of the increases in tumors were seen in people over seventy, who actually had the least exposure to aspartame. There is no evidence to support that aspartame is the cause of increases in cancer.

But, as with vaccines and autism, once the myth is out there, the truth is hard to swallow. People started to blame their headaches on aspartame, even though a randomized, double-blinded, placebo-controlled study showed that aspartame did not cause headaches in "aspartame sensitive" people. Others started to claim that sodas with aspartame were high in methanol. Analyses show that there is more methanol in a glass of tomato juice, or in fruits and vegetables, than in a diet soda. Another randomized double-blinded, placebo-controlled study (a great study!) showed that aspartame had no effect on mood, memory, behavior, EEG results, or physiology. And, finally, a prospective study of 285,079 men and 188,905 women ages fifty to seventy-one in the NIH-AARP Diet and Health Study could detect no effect of aspartame consumption on the development of blood or brain cancers.

There's just no evidence. In study after study, these artificial sweeteners have not been shown to be the health risks that many make them out to be. It's a myth.

Bathroom

The door handle is the dirtiest fixture in the bathroom

One thing we hear all the time from friends and family is the lengths they will go not to touch things in the restroom. One of the most common strategies involves using a paper towel to open the bathroom door. People seem to be genuinely afraid of the door handle. Rachel recently heard a woman pushing a public bathroom door open with her elbow repeatedly say "touching the door handle in a bathroom will make you sick." Once Rachel left the bathroom, she saw that same woman smoking. Hmm. That's interesting.

Let's take a breather and think this through. It's important to think about why we assume certain things are "dirty" or can harbor infection. In the case of the bathroom, it's because we know something "dirty" occurs there. Picture a bathroom in your head. We bet you didn't picture a sparkling clean room, shiny and bright. We bet you pictured a dark, dank, filthy room. But it's important to remember that that's your impression. It's not necessarily based on fact.

The truth is that the actual dirtiness of an object or place comes down to two factors: (1) how many people have touched it with dirty hands, and (2) how often it is cleaned. With respect to the door handle of the bathroom, we can't vouch for (2), but we bet it's more often than the door handle in your office. But here's the thing, as for (1), the door handle in the bathroom is touched far more often by clean hands—they've just been washed—than dirty.

In fact, the door handle seems to be one of the cleanest things in the bathroom. Don't take our word for it; it's been studied. Dr. Chuck Gerba, known also as "Dr. Germ," has conducted a number of studies in this area. Someone had to, we guess. In one study, he found that toilet seats and door handles are the cleanest surfaces in public bathrooms. Amazing, but true! The bathroom floor was the dirtiest thing in the bathroom by a long shot, and often contained more than two million bacteria per square inch. So don't put your purse or briefcase on the floor (which we bet lots of you do)!

Faucets and sinks are also worse than the door handles or toilets. That's because people don't wash their hands before touching those. Again, this has been studied. It's not our guess. Think back to those rules we mentioned before. Think about the many things that are touched by lots of dirty hands and never cleaned. Things like elevator buttons. Shopping carts. Money machine buttons. Supermarket self-serve checkout machines. Playground equipment. Hotel room remotes.

Should we continue?

We don't say this to make you crazy. After all, many of you are touching these things all the time and will not get sick as a result.

Air dryers will keep your hands cleaner than paper towels

One of the best things about writing a book like this is that we get to discover some amazing science being done by people we would never otherwise hear of. One of those people is Dr. Keith Redway of the School of Biomedical Sciences at the University of Westminster in London. Believe us when we tell you that he is the man when it comes to drying your hands in the bathroom. Sure, other people have done some work in the area, but no one else—to our knowledge—has dedicated himself to the truly important question of how best to dry your hands in a public restroom. Don't take our word for it. Go look him up.

Why is Dr. Redway's work important? Well, how many times have you finished washing your hands at the sink and been presented with the impossible choice of whether to use the hot air dryer or paper towels? From what we see online and hear from many of you, the overwhelming choice would be to use the air dryer. People believe it's more sanitary than paper towels. After all, you need to touch nothing to use it. Many air dryers even have claims about being more sanitary printed right on the machine.

But is that true? In a series of experiments, Dr. Redway and a colleague of his decided to find out. For each of these studies, they compared different paper towels, warm air dryers, and newer jet air dryers.

First, they looked at how well each of these methods achieved dryness. After all, that is the primary purpose of drying your hands. Specifically, they measured the amount of water remaining on the hands at different times up to one minute. They found that all five types of paper towels and the jet air dryer achieved 90 percent dryness by ten seconds. The warm air dryer took much longer to achieve the same effect. Make of that what you will.

The next study was where it gets interesting. How much does using each of these drying mechanisms affect germs on your hands? They took twenty people and measured the numbers and types of bacteria on their hands both before and after using two types of paper towels and the warm air and jet air dryer. Both types of paper towels reduced the number of all types of bacteria on both the palms and fingertips. Warm air dryers, on the other hand, actually increased the number of all types of bacteria and the jet air dryer increased the number of most types of bacteria on both the palms and fingertips. The paper towels were the obvious winners in terms of reducing bacteria on hands.

But they weren't done yet. For their next study, they took ten people and artificially contaminated their hands with a yeast suspension. Again, they had them dry with two types of paper towels and the warm air and jet air dryer. The point of this was to see how these drying methods contaminated the rest of the environment. They found that the jet air dryer dispersed the contaminant over two meters from where the dryer was located. The warm air dryer was slightly worse than the paper towels in that it dispersed more contaminant, but only directly below the dryer.

There's more. In a final experiment, they went to sixteen public restrooms in a London rail station and swabbed the jet air dryers to see what kind of bacteria was there to be potentially spread around the room and onto hands. They also measured what was contained in air emitted from them over a ten-second period. They found a large number of bacteria, some of which were potential pathogens.

So to sum it up, paper towels dried just as well as anything, removed more bacteria that were on the hands already, and did not contaminate other parts of the bathroom. Seems like an easy decision on which to use next time.

We should note that other work has been done comparing air dryers to paper towels. Some of the work agrees with Dr. Redway's findings. Some of it finds less of a difference between the methods. We should also note that Dr. Redway has often been funded by the paper towel industry in his research. But we can find no fault with his methods, and no one seems to have the single-mindedness of his calling.

The idea that hot air or jet air dryers are superior (in cleanliness or drying ability) is simply a myth.

Bubbles

The bubbles in soda will make
your bones brittle

There are plenty of arguments to be made about the negative nutritional effects of soda, especially nondiet soda, which is full of empty sugar calories. One thing about soda that is not harmful, though, is its carbonation. In spite of this, many people believe that the bubbles in soda will negatively affect your bone structure.

This belief can be blamed, in part, on misunderstanding some studies from the turn of this century. A study published in the *American Journal of Clinical Nutrition* found that excess urinary excretion of calcium occurred when people drank carbonated drinks with caffeine. That means that people drinking carbonated, caffeinated drinks were peeing out more calcium. However, this study also noted that, later in the day, the kidneys compensated by lowering the amount of calcium excreted in the urine. This meant the overall loss of calcium was negligible. They concluded that the seemingly negative bone health effects of drinking carbonated beverages were likely due to the fact that people drinking soda were less likely to drink milk. Since this research was funded in part by Dairy Management, Inc., a significant conflict of interest exists.

There is some evidence that carbonated cola drinks might have some connection with weaker bones. Another study was conducted by scientists at Tufts University. They looked at data from 2,500 women and men (ages forty-nine to sixty-nine) who took part in the Framingham Osteoporosis Study. They found that noncola carbonated drinks were not associated with low bone mineral density; cola intake, on the other hand, was associated with lower bone mineral density at the hip in women, but not in men, and in neither group's spines. There was a dose response, in that women who drank more cola had more of an effect. Contradicting the theorizing at the end of the study, women who drank more cola did not drink less milk, although their overall intake of calcium was lower. This study offers some suggestion that there might be a tie between weaker bones and cola, but not with carbonation.

Backing this up is an additional study published in the *British Journal of Nutrition* in 2005. Researchers gathered a group of otherwise healthy women who had gone through menopause and compared those who drank noncarbonated mineral water to those who drank carbonated mineral water. Specifically, they looked at whether tests of blood and urine could detect changes in bone turnover, a sign of bone weakening. They could detect no differences after eight weeks. The carbonation alone clearly does not make a difference.

Even the studies that came out against soda in some way focus on colas. None specifically implicates carbonation. There seem to be no problems with sparkling mineral water or seltzer. The carbonation is not to blame for any bone mineral problems or for low levels of calcium. And even if you think caffeine or other things in colas might take away your body's calcium, go ahead and make sure to get enough calcium from other sources. But don't worry about the bubbles. They won't do you any harm.

Caffeine

Caffeine stunts your growth

Aaron loves coffee. Loves it. In fact, he's somewhat of a coffee nut and has been known to roast his own beans. But when he was young, his parents—like many of yours—told him that he couldn't drink coffee because it would stunt his growth. That was the line in Rachel's family too, but since they were all tall Dutch people who had consumed massive amounts of coffee from young ages, the threat didn't hold much credence.

It's not totally clear where this myth comes from. Ironically, some believe it stems from the same literature that allegedly linked carbonation to brittle bones. If you remember, those studies found that it wasn't the bubbles in the drink, but perhaps the caffeine that led to problems in calcium in bones. Some people may have extrapolated this to mean that caffeine reduces the calcium available to your bones, which leads to bone problems, which leads to stunted growth. Case closed!

Or not. When we follow coffee or caffeine drinkers over time in good prospective studies, we see that this really isn't the case. Growing bones does require your body to use calcium. If caffeine prevents your body from absorbing calcium, then it seems feasible that caffeine would stunt bone growth. Science does not bear this out. In studies, caffeine did slightly limit how well the gut absorbed calcium. However, the studies also showed that the body compensates easily for this change in calcium absorption, by decreasing how much calcium it gets rid of in your pee over a twenty-four-hour period. The overall difference in calcium absorption is quite small. In fact, the study finding that calcium was not absorbed as well when you drink caffeine stated that whatever negative effects the caffeine had on calcium absorption could be overcome by drinking an extra one or two tablespoons of milk.

Some posit that people who drink caffeine may be taking in less dairy or drinking less milk. That's possible, but it's a far cry from claiming that coffee stunts your growth.

There's more. Another study enrolled eighty-one girls between ages twelve to eighteen to see how caffeine affected their total body bone mineral gain and hip bone density over a six-year period. One group consumed less than 25 mg of caffeine per day, one consumed 25 to 50 mg of caffeine per day, and one consumed greater than 50 mg of caffeine per day. The researchers found that there were no significant differences among the three groups with respect to the bone health. Caffeine intake at various levels did not affect bone health or growth.

Caffeine is a commonly used drug in the neonatal intensive care unit, where premature babies are cared for. We use it to stimulate them when their brains are immature; it helps them to breathe on their own. If there was any real evidence that caffeine would stunt their growth, we wouldn't be using it there.

There are, of course, plenty of reasons not to give kids caffeine. Unlike sugar, caffeine can affect their behavior and even their sleep. But it won't stunt their growth.

Cancer

Cancer is unpreventable

Cancer is scary. Many people don't like to talk about it at all because they fear it so much. A lot of the fear comes from a belief that there's nothing you can do to prevent cancer. That's totally not true. And getting over this myth could actually save your life.

First of all, there are a number of things that people do that seriously increase their risk of getting cancer. Our advice: stop doing them. For instance, tobacco use is significantly associated with cancers of all types. The scary truth is that smoking cigarettes has been proven to be associated with cancer in the lungs, mouth, throat, kidney, bladder, stomach, pancreas, and cervix. It can also cause certain types of leukemia. Studies have shown that about 30 percent of all cancer deaths occurring in the United States are caused by smoking cigarettes. Don't do it. Not smoking in the first place or quitting smoking if you do is probably the very best way to prevent cancer.

Another major cause of cancer is infection. Luckily, many of these infections are also preventable. For instance, human papillomavirus (HPV) is well established as the cause for cervical cancer. Luckily, there is now a vaccine for HPV, which can lead to a significant decrease in precancerous lesions. A vaccine to protect people against cancer is a great thing! Hepatitis B is also known to lead to liver cancers. There's a vaccine for that too. Granted, some viruses that lead to cancer can't be prevented by vaccine, but many types of cancer can be avoided by taking good care of your body.

Radiation exposure can also lead to cancer. Specifically, ultraviolet radiation from the sun is a major cause of skin cancer. So, cover up, or at least use sunblock. Ionizing radiation is even more of a concern in regard to cancer, because it actually rips electrons from their orbit, killing or irreparably harming components of some of your body's cells. These cells can then go on to become cancer. Ionizing radiation can come from either medical sources, such as radiological scans, or from radon in homes. Most of the increase in radiation exposure in recent years is because of the increased use of CT scans in medical practice. Try to avoid these when you can.

There are a number of other things you can do to prevent cancer, although there is not as much evidence for them compared to what we've already discussed. A number of reviews have been conducted, and most point to the fact that fruits and nonstarchy vegetables are associated with a decrease in the risk of getting cancer. However, when these types of food are carefully studied in scientific randomized controlled trials, their protective effects are not clearly seen. Similarly, alcohol has been linked to some cancers. But no conclusive evidence exists. Since we always rely on evidence to make declarative statements, we can say with confidence that a diet high in fruits and nonstarchy vegetables, without alcohol abuse, may reduce your risk of cancer and definitely will result in better overall health.

Lots of people will tell you that vitamin and mineral supplements will prevent cancer. This, unfortunately, goes over the line into the myth category itself. No good evidence exists that they do any good. In fact, a prospective study of beta-carotene (vitamin A) found that it might actually increase your risk of lung cancer. Antioxidants like vitamin E or selenium have failed to show any significant results in studies. Vitamins C and E do not prevent prostate cancer. And the Women's Antioxidant Cardiovascular Study could detect no protective effects for vitamins C, E, B$_6$, B$_{12}$, folic acid, or beta-carotene.

The problem with all this is that we often pin false hopes on things that don't work and ignore the obvious things that do. It would be great if popping a few vitamin pills would prevent cancer. But they won't. What will is avoiding tobacco and the sun, getting necessary vaccines, and, perhaps, eating more healthily.

Celery

Celery has negative calories

The key to weight loss or weight gain is simple: it is all a matter of how many calories you take in and how many calories you burn. If you burn more calories than you take in, then you will lose weight. If you burn the same number of calories as you take in, then you will maintain the same weight. In this equation, celery has come to hold a legendary role among dieters. In contrast to most foods, which add to the calories you take in, celery is reported to have "negative calories." The idea is that you use up more calories in the act of eating the celery than are actually contained in the vegetable.

It is true that celery can be a great part of your diet when you're trying to lose weight. An eight-inch stalk of celery contains only six calories. Not much at all, but it does contain *some* calories. Do we use up that many calories chewing up the celery? Probably not. The body burns roughly eighty-five calories per hour while eating (not so much more than the sixty calories per hour it uses when you are sleeping!). This means that in one minute of eating, you only use up 1.4 calories. It would have to take you several minutes of chewing to burn up the number of calories in a stick of celery, and even though those stringy stalks take some time, it probably does not take you four minutes to chew one piece.

However, you just might use up all those calories in the stick of celery from the process of digesting the celery. Much of celery is a substance called cellulose that the human body does not digest, and which passes through our system without being absorbed. Cellulose is not metabolized by humans, and so your body needs to pass it through to the other end. In the much longer time needed to pass that celery through your system, your body will have used more than the six calories in that piece of celery.

Does this mean that the celery will help you lose weight? Not necessarily. In order to lose a pound of body weight, you need to take in about 3,500 calories fewer than you use up. The six calories in celery and the small calorie deficit that you might get from your body digesting the celery are a far cry from 3,500 net calories used up. And in case you have heard that celery is a special negative calorie food that somehow boosts your metabolism and makes you burn other foods up faster, you should know that there is absolutely no evidence for this. So, the point we're trying to make here is quite simple: there is nothing magical about celery. Losing weight still requires you to take in fewer calories than you burn. Celery might help you toward your goal, but it is likely to play only a very small role.

Cell Phones

Cell phones cause brain tumors

Let's start with some facts. Cell phones are hugely popular. Worldwide estimates put their usage at more than three billion people. In the United States, more than 270 million people use cell phones, including about half of children age eight to twelve. We also know that exposure to radiation increases your risk of developing cancer (see the section on cancer). And cell phones do emit radiation. So it shouldn't come as a surprise that there is an ongoing debate as to whether this widespread use of a device that emits radiation causes cancer—specifically brain tumors.

Many studies have been published in this area. The vast majority of them are what we call case-control studies: First, you gather a group of people with brain tumors. Then, you gather a group of people without brain tumors. Then you ask them about their day-to-day activities (such as the frequency of cell phone use) to see if there are differences between the two groups.

While this type of study can sometimes give us good information, it's important to recognize that case-control studies are among the weaker types of scientific studies. Unlike randomized controlled trials, a case-control study will not prove that cell phones do or do not cause brain tumors. And, unlike in prospective cohort studies, which follow a group of people forward in time through the study, there is a real problem with recall bias. Recall bias happens when someone with a particular issue or disease (in this case, a brain tumor) is more likely to recall activities that might have caused their issue or disease than someone who does not. The danger with case-control studies is that people with brain tumors may have heard the theory that cell phones cause brain tumors, and therefore may be more apt to recall their cell phone use than people without brain tumors.

There are so many of these studies about cell phones that we won't try to summarize them all. Luckily, that has already been done for us! In 2008, a scientist summarized data from thirty-three studies in the peer-reviewed scientific literature. This summary found major flaws in the research that make it difficult to draw solid conclusions from all of these studies.

Another group attempted a meta-analysis of the literature. They felt that twenty-three studies were good enough to be included in the analysis. All of them were case-control studies. They found overall that, compared to rarely or never using a cell phone, regularly using a cell phone did not cause malignant or benign brain tumors.

The studies point out some important issues contradicting the idea that cell phone use is connected to brain tumors: With so many people using cell phones, you could expect, if there was a major association between cell phones and brain tumors, the number of tumors would be through the roof. Three billion people use cell phones! Even if there is an association, it has to be very small. Moreover, the types of brain tumors that have been more common recently take decades to appear. Cell phones, on the other hand, are a relatively new invention. We know from previous work that there is usually a long time period between exposure to radiation and the development of slow-growing brain tumors. According to that timeline, even if there were a link, we shouldn't see a jump in brain tumors caused by cell phones until the 2030s.

Let's remember something else too: there are much greater risks to our lives than cell phones. That's for sure. After all, the number one killer of children in the U.S. is car accidents, and yet how many people out there think cars should be banned? As a society, we accept that the quality of life derived from driving is greater than the risks having people die in car accidents. If you disagree, don't drive. Almost no one does that. The risk of brain tumors is so low that, even if it exists, few would likely forgo their cell phone to reduce it.

Furthermore, although we talk about an increase in brain tumors, there has been no explosion of brain tumors recently in the population. A study published in the *Journal of the National Cancer Institute* in 2009 examined data for cancers in four countries with registries from 1974 to 2003. Over that time, almost 60,000 people in a population of 16 million adults between ten and seventy-nine years were diagnosed with brain tumors. While a slow increase in rates of gliomas and meningiomas (faster-growing tumors) was seen throughout the same time period, no changes in incidence were seen from 1998 to 2003, five years when cell phone use increased dramatically and when you would expect to see more brain tumors because of that increase.

Case-control studies are a reasonable measure for determining a link between the activities we undertake and the diseases we develop. But cell phones are so widely used that, honestly, if they were so dangerous, we'd be seeing that effect right now. That's just not happening. Additional studies will be needed to see if they cause long-term harm, but as of now, this is a myth.

Cheese

Cheese makes you constipated

If you want to consider foods that get an unfair shake, it's worth talking about cheese. Aaron's son Noah loves cheese. He loves it almost as much as chicken nuggets and fries, which he would eat for three meals a day, seven days a week if permitted. It's all part of his "beige food" diet, which someday he will turn into fame and fortune. Anyway, Aaron has been guilty of putting strict limits on Noah's cheese intake because he, like many of you, has been told that cheese causes constipation. But is it true?

If you go to any number of Web sites dedicated to constipation, it sure seems like it's true. (By the way, why are there so many Web sites dedicated to constipation?) These sites will tell you that both a low-fiber diet and too much dairy consumption (especially cheese), will lead to constipation.

But the science behind all of this is not nearly so cut-and-dry. The belief that dairy products cause constipation was born mostly from studies of constipation in babies. Parents are obsessed with babies' pooping, as we detailed in our last book. So much so that parents constantly bring their children to the doctor to talk about the child's poop. Constipation is the reason for about one in four visits to pediatric gastroenterology clinics. But baby constipation and childhood or adult constipation are two different issues.

If you look at the data from babies, there is some connection between dairy intake and firmer stools or constipation. The proteins in breast milk are easily digested, as they are designed to be.

However, the proteins in baby formula are not the same as those in breast milk, and the proteins in formula most often come from cow's milk. Infants who are fed formula (which is cow's milk–based) have firmer stools and more frequently have problems with constipation. Other factors, like fat content, can also affect the consistency of infant stools.

But there are many problems with simply extrapolating this data about cow's milk formula and applying it to children and adults. First of all, a lot of what those parents think is constipation is not really constipation. Second, the issues infants might have with cow's milk formula are not the same as children or adults might have with cheese. They aren't the same at all.

Some people have digestive issues with milk or dairy. Those issues are real. But they also usually have more to do with diarrhea, bloating, or discomfort—not constipation. Lactose intolerance, in which people cannot digest the sugar called lactose found in dairy products, generally makes your stool loose and you gassy, not constipated. In fact, a study of people who reported sensitivity to dairy products did find an association between exposure to cow's milk and increased immune system activation (with more immunoglobulins present), but the study found no statistically significant association with constipation. Even people who were sensitive to cow's milk did not have any issues with constipation from dairy products.

There are very few good studies examining the relationship between cheese and constipation. But there is one particularly strong study. The National Health and Nutrition Examination Survey (NHANES) was put together by the National Center for Health Statistics in 1971–1975. They gathered tons of data on diet, exercise, and bowel dysfunction (among other data). In 1990, a group of researchers looked at data from the study for over 15,000 people age twelve to seventy-four. Overall, just under 13 percent of people reported constipation. When they did analyses on what those people were eating, constipated people reported eating less cheese, not more. They also ate less beans and peas, less milk, less meat and chicken, and less fruits and vegetables. They also drank more coffee and tea.

We're not suggesting that diet has nothing to do with constipation. We're also not suggesting that there aren't people who have dairy issues. But no good evidence exists to implicate cheese in causing constipation in otherwise healthy people, and what evidence does exist, actually points the other way. Noah is going to be so pleased.

Chicken Soup

I have just the thing for that cold . . .
Chicken Soup—TRUE

As myth busters, it's sort of our job to dispel a lot of the "wisdom" that your mother and grandmother swore by. But one of Grandma's best remedies may actually have something to offer when it comes to treating your cold. Yes, chicken soup might actually help relieve your cold symptoms.

We have to start off by saying that chicken soup has not been tested in rigorous, clinical studies. The evidence for or against chicken soup is not up to the standards of the studies that show us that medicines like antihistamines do not work for colds. However, experts have proposed several ways that chicken soup might work to help your body fight a cold or feel better during a cold. Chicken soup is a source of hydration and may improve your nutritional status: both good boosts when you are sick. The warm liquid may also help you better clear mucus from your body, especially from your nose. In a study that compared the impact of drinking hot water, cold water, and chicken soup, both hot water and chicken soup increased how fast the nose was running or helped to clear out the nose, but the chicken soup worked even better than the hot water alone.

It is also possible that chicken soup could have some special ability to kill cells involved with infections. And some experts have proposed that chicken soup might make you feel better by lessening your body's inflammatory response to an infection, so that you don't have as much mucus or as many aches and pains.

As mentioned, chicken soup has not been studied very rigorously in groups of sick or healthy people, but one group of researchers did carefully investigate the impact of chicken soup on the specific cells of the immune system that increase inflammation when you have an infection. When you have an infection, immune cells called neutrophils migrate to the area to help fight the infection. One of the things those neutrophils do is release chemicals that increase the amount of inflammation going on in your body. This inflammation is part of why you develop more mucus and phlegm when you have a cold. Though some of the inflammation response helps to fight off infection, other aspects of inflammation make you feel lousy.

Scientists studied whether chicken soup had an impact on the inflammation response. The scientists studied a homemade chicken soup, as well as commercially prepared soups, to determine whether chicken soup prevented the inflammatory cells from migrating or moving to the source of infection. Amazingly enough, chicken soup worked! Various dilutions of the homemade soup and the majority of the store-bought soups inhibited the movement of the neutrophil cells, which might give chicken soup anti-inflammatory properties.

Chicken soup is not proven to be an effective cold remedy, but it does have some properties that might help you feel a bit better. You may also experience the best kind of placebo effect from chicken soup. Having soup prepared for you by a loved one, or associating chicken soup with memories of someone taking good care of you, may play a powerful role in how much better chicken soup helps you to feel. Chicken soup is not the cure for the common cold, but the science suggests that it may be worthwhile to listen to Grandma on this one. You just might feel a bit better.

Chocolate

Chocolate or fried foods cause acne

Those of us with acne will try almost anything to improve our skin. Everyone wants clear skin. When you have pimples popping up all over, your parents and other well-meaning people often tell you to avoid chocolate or fried foods because these foods make acne worse. Many acne sufferers swear that they see differences in how bad their acne is based on what they eat. Whether or not your diet will sabotage your efforts to have clear skin is a question addressed by some interesting science.

Studies show us that people around the world believe that there is some link between acne and what they eat. The belief that particular foods make acne worse has been reported in studies of acne sufferers and their families from countries ranging from Greece to Britain to Jordan. Greasy food is most often reported as a cause of acne, perhaps reflecting beliefs that greasy skin and eating greasy food are linked. Nonmedical people are not the only ones who are not sure what makes acne better or worse; medical students, nurses, and family practice doctors have also been shown to have very limited knowledge about what worsens acne and what works to treat it.

The science about acne and what we eat is actually rather tricky to sort through. A number of studies have looked at how many people suffer from acne in different parts of the world. These studies find that acne is more common among adolescents in places like the United States and Canada than it is in certain parts of Africa or in other isolated places, like Papua New Guinea or among certain groups in Paraguay or Brazil. The low rates of acne in places where people are eating very different foods than we do in America make scientists wonder whether your diet really does make a difference for your acne. People in America and Canada do eat more chocolate and more fried, greasy foods than people in these other places. The problem with these studies is that other factors could also be making a difference in the rates of acne. Certain ethnic groups might just be less prone to developing acne. Or other factors related to the environment or skin care practices might play a role. The studies of how common acne is in certain places do not actually tell us that foods are to blame, and they definitely don't tell us which foods might be to blame.

To try to find out whether certain foods are to blame, other scientists have tried to look more specifically at what people eat and whether they have acne. (Rachel really just cares about chocolate, so that is the one we will look at most carefully.) Chocolate, fried or greasy foods, and foods with a lot of sugar are often blamed for causing acne or for making your breakouts worse. We have often heard this debunked as a myth, but it took some research to look at all the evidence. Scientists have often tested these foods in regard to acne by testing whether the foods increase insulin resistance. Insulin is a particular hormone that helps the body absorb sugars, but it is also involved in a sequence of hormone responses in your body that has been linked to how we develop acne. Your body's reaction to insulin can actually impact the other hormones, like androgens and retinoids, that are more directly linked to developing acne. Scientists have speculated that foods that make you more resistant to insulin might also give you more acne by increasing these other hormones. While studies of animals have almost always shown that foods with lots of fats (like chocolate or fried foods) increase the body's resistance to insulin, many of the studies in humans have not found such a link between eating a lot of fat and having more insulin resistance. There is also no evidence that eating a lot of sugar (or having high glycemic indexes) makes humans have too much insulin or makes them resistant to insulin in ways that would cause acne. Whether or not eating a lot of fat or sugar changes the body's resistance to insulin has important implications for problems like diabetes and obesity. Scientists need to do more work to figure out whether or how these foods impact the body's long-term response to insulin. In the meantime, there is not definitive evidence that high-fat or high-sugar foods will increase insulin resistance in a way that causes you to have more acne.

The other hypothesis that scientists have tested is whether foods with more fat or sugar might increase how much sebum comes out of your pores. Sebum is basically what makes your skin oily, the natural oil of the skin. It is trapped sebum in the pores of your skin that gets inflamed and causes acne. Do fatty foods increase how much sebum you are making? Once again, some of the studies in animals show that animals do make more sebum when they eat more fat. In human studies, there is some suggestion that what you eat might change the amount of sebum your skin makes and how much fat is in that sebum. However, the human studies do not show that this change in the sebum impacts your acne.

Two studies have specifically tested whether chocolate impacts acne in humans. The studies did not have huge numbers of volunteers and were not designed as well as we would have liked, but both studies did not show any connection between chocolate and acne. In one of the studies, volunteers were given either chocolate bars or a fake chocolate bar that had similar amounts of fat and sugar. Those who were given the actual chocolate bars did not have any more acne, did not make any more sebum (skin oil), and did not have any changes in the composition of their sebum when they were compared to those eating the placebo bars. Several other small studies that asked people about their diets and about their acne found no connection between having acne and how much sugar they eat, how much chocolate they eat, shellfish, sweets, pizza, French fries, or other fatty foods.

A number of people have also questioned whether milk was to blame for acne breakouts. Because most chocolate contains milk, if milk is to blame for acne problems, this could also implicate chocolate. In several small studies, researchers have not found any connection between how much milk or other dairy products people eat and whether they have more acne. However, in a big study of thousands of nurses, there was an association between those who reported a history of having acne as a teenager and those who reported drinking more milk as a teenager. Scientists have come up with lots of theories as to why milk might cause more acne. In particular, they have speculated that hormones or other substances like iodine in the milk might make adolescents' acne worse. These theories sound like they might make sense, but they haven't been proven. And even the big study that connected milk intake and acne has some serious flaws. First of all, this kind of connection is an association, not causation. There is no proof that the milk *causes* the acne; the linkage can only say that they are correlated. Second, the data in the study relies on people's memories of what they ate or drank. In comes the potential problem of recall bias that we have talked about before. It is very possible that if you had a problem like acne and you thought that milk might be involved, you would remember your milk-drinking more clearly than people who never had issues with acne.

Even though people all around the world believe that their diet affects their acne, there is no good scientific evidence that this is the case. Experts have developed ideas about how certain foods might make acne worse, but the scientific tests of these ideas let the foods off the hook! Both chocolate and fatty foods have been studied, and are not linked to acne. As is often the case, though, it would be great to have bigger and better studies to try to help us understand what really does make pimples pop up. In summary, there is no good scientific evidence to suggest that chocolate or fried foods are to blame for making your acne worse. A healthy diet should only include chocolate or fried foods in moderation; you can certainly enjoy these treats occasionally without pimple paranoia.

Cold Weather

Cold weather (and being underdressed for cold weather) will make you sick

Does the cold give you a cold? Around the world, people believe that cold or wet weather makes you sick. "If you go out in the cold or get too cold, you will catch a cold!" warn mothers and grandmothers everywhere. In studies from around the world, people report more colds when they are in cold, wet conditions. When Rachel is in Kenya, a country in East Africa that is directly on the equator, it is quite a bit warmer than in the middle of the United States where Aaron spends most his time; but if the temperature in Kenya drops just a little bit, everyone expects that they will get sick quickly because of the "cold." Parents in the United States have the same fears as parents in Kenya. Sixty percent of American parents in one survey believed that changes in the weather cause colds, and 38 percent believed that cold weather causes colds. Just over half of the parents thought that not wearing enough clothes could cause a cold too. These were not poorly educated parents either; 48 percent had gone to some college or graduated from college, and an additional 35 percent had gone to graduate school.

Should we believe all of these reports of getting sick more often when it is cold? Not necessarily. When the question is studied scientifically, the answer is often quite different. Back in the 1930s, scientists studied the inhabitants of a small, freezing-cold island in the Arctic Sea to see how often they got sick. While they may have been bored on their cold little island, these islanders were not getting sick because of it. Scientists did not find any cases of colds during the winter, and the island inhabitants only started getting sick when the weather warmed up and outside ships brought in other people (including some with colds).

Colds are not caused by the weather; they are caused by something that human beings pass from one to another. Colds are caused by rhinoviruses—a particularly unpleasant family of very similar viruses that cause runny noses, scratchy, sore throats, and general cold-related misery. With so many slightly different varieties, there are enough cold viruses to keep you getting sick again and again over the course of your life, without ever building up immunity to every single one. A new one can always come along and make you miserable with a cold once again.

Even if it is the virus that makes you sick, you might still believe the cold weather plays a role in getting that virus. Does the cold hurt our immune systems and make us more susceptible to getting sick? Actually, the opposite seems to be true. In a study of how the body's immune system reacts to cold exposure, the researchers actually found that the immune system was stimulated when people were exposed to the cold. The cold weather increased the number and the activity level of some of the body's key sickness-fighting cells—the white blood cells (specifically, the leukocytes and the granulocytes for those of you who want to look for them under a microscope). Other chemicals that the body produces to fight infections were also increased. So, the cold weather actually may help your body to fight sickness! In this study, the researchers also looked at what would happen if you were warmed up first or exercised before your cold exposure. As it turns out, getting warmed up before you go out into the cold helps your immune system work even better. The infection-fighting cells and substances in your body increase even more if you are warmed up before you go out into the cold.

Even though your body may have better sickness-fighting ability during the cold weather, it still seems like people get sick more often when it is cold outside, especially during the wintertime. The cause of the seasonality of colds (known to doctors as upper respiratory tract infections) is not entirely clear. One explanation is that people spend more time indoors when it is cold outside, staying in relatively close proximity to one another and allowing them to pass those colds around with their sneezing and coughing. Another idea that one expert suggests is that cold weather keeps the airways in your nose cooler, and this decrease in the temperature of the inside of your nose gets in the way of how the nose works to protect you from colds. Even though the rest of the body's immune system seems to be activated by the cold weather, when the nose is exposed to cold temperatures, the tiny hairs and mucus that keep things moving out of your nose might not work as well. This could give the cold viruses a chance to settle in and make you sick. While these studies show how the cold theoretically hinders how well your nose works to protect you, there is not yet wide-scale evidence that this is the reason people get sick in the wintertime.

There is a cycle of when certain viruses come and go. The rhinoviruses that cause most colds actually peak in the spring and fall, perhaps contributing to the belief that we get sick when the weather changes. Other families of viruses peak in the winter—viruses like those of the influenza family, which usually cause the much worse flu, or respiratory syncytial virus (RSV), which can make babies very sick and usually cause a cold in adults. We do not have a good explanation for why particular parts of the world see these viruses at particular times, but it is not necessarily the cold weather that brings them around. Don't blame Frosty!

Plus, it is important to remember that the practical effects of cold exposure on getting sick have been tested. When scientists test what the cold virus does in humans, there is no evidence that the cold weather makes you more susceptible to infection. In study after study where scientists put cold viruses directly into people's noses and then measure who gets infected, the people who are forced to be in very cold conditions are no more likely to get infected with a cold than the people who got to stay in warm conditions.

Researchers have even studied the question of whether or not wearing enough clothes when it is cold will make you get sick. In one study, volunteers were divided into groups where some people had to be in very cold conditions, but were allowed to wear warm coats; others had to be in their underwear in 60 degree temperatures; and a third group got to be the lucky ones in 80 degrees of warmth. It turns out that it didn't matter at all how cold it was or what you were wearing; everyone with the virus stuck into their nose had the same risk of getting infected by that virus.

There has been one study that suggested that if a particular body part got very chilled, you were more likely to report experiencing cold symptoms. In this study, all of the volunteers were again exposed to the cold virus, and then some of them had to keep their feet in very cold water. Those who had chilled feet were more likely to report cold symptoms later on. Does this mean that you better make sure you are wearing warm socks and boots? While having cozy feet is always nice, it won't necessarily affect whether you get sick. This study could not establish a cause-and-effect relationship. While icy toes and having a runny nose might be linked in some way, it could be that you just notice your runny nose more because you remember how cold your feet were and have been terrified about getting sick. There is no evidence to prove you are more likely to get a cold from leaving a body part without warm enough socks or gloves.

What about wearing a hat? Your mother may have convinced you that the reason the cold weather was finally going to make you sick was because you did not cover your head. Many people have heard that covering your head is the most important thing you can do to stay warm since you lose the majority of your body heat through your head. This is a myth, too! You do lose body heat through your head, but you lose heat through any part of your body that is uncovered. The amount of heat loss depends on the surface area of what is uncovered. You don't lose any more heat from your uncovered head than you do from an uncovered arm or an uncovered leg. The one thing that is special about the head is how we feel about heat when our heads are covered or uncovered. Studies have shown that how warm people feel when their head is covered is out of proportion with how warm they actually are. "Thermal sensation," or feeling warm, is increased when you wear a hat more than your actual body heat is increased. Along with the studies examining whether people who are not dressed warmly enough get sick, scientists have studied whether cold viruses will infect you if you are not wearing a hat. However, bald people do not become sick more easily than people with hair. There is no evidence that people who go without hats get sick more often. Similarly, there is no evidence linking baldness (where your head is always less covered) with any sicknesses except sunburn and potentially skin cancer.

If you are cold and your head is still uncovered, then by all means put on a hat! But a hat alone is not a guarantee of warmth or health. You may be tempted to stay inside or wear extra layers of clothes when it is cold outside. There is certainly nothing wrong with being comfortable, but you should be reasonable about why you take your precautions. The cold weather may make you uncomfortable, but it is not going to make you sick.

Cough and Cold Medicines

I have just the thing for that cold . . .
Over-the-Counter Cough and Cold Medicines

When you are suffering from a terrible cold, that long aisle at the drugstore with its myriad cough and cold remedies appears promising. The various pills and syrups promise to improve your stuffed-up or runny nose, your hacking cough, your scratchy throat, or all of the above. Yes, please! But you may find it hard to know which one will work best. What might be even harder to grasp is that none of these medicines will actually cure your cold. Colds and coughs are almost always caused by viruses, and none of the medicines on the drugstore shelf are designed to kill viruses. Instead, they are supposed to help with your symptoms, such as making your nose run less or relieving your congestion.

Antihistamines are one type of medicine commonly used to treat the symptoms of the common cold. When scientists looked at combined results from thirty-two studies of antihistamines involving almost 9,000 people, they do not find any improvement overall from using an antihistamine by itself for either children or adults. In the small subset of patients who did report some improvement after taking an antihistamine, 81 percent of the patients still had cold symptoms even with this improvement. For children, antihistamines did not perform any better than a placebo in any of the studies.

Many over-the-counter cough and cold medicines are combined medicines that include both an antihistamine and a decongestant. In studies involving children, these combined antihistamines and decongestants did not have any effect; they simply did not improve cold symptoms for children under five. For older children and adults, though, there was a small benefit. Similarly, decongestants alone seem to have some benefit for patients with colds. So, if you want to improve your nasal stuffiness or congestion, a combined antihistamine and decongestant or a decongestant alone might help you, but an antihistamine alone will not make a difference.

Some studies have shown that nasal sprays can relieve congestion for approximately one day, but there is no evidence that using them again and again will help you. In fact, many people develop a "rebound" runny nose or congestion when they use these nasal decongestants for more than one or two days.

When it comes to medicines that relieve your cough (antitussives), we again find that most do not work when you look at the science. A review of studies evaluating what helps or does not help with coughs in adults found that codeine did not help with coughs any more than a placebo or fake medicine did. Another common anti-coughing medicine called moguisteine did not work either. There was some evidence that a medicine called dextromethorphan (you see this in medicines labeled "DM") did help with coughs; two of the studies showed that dextromethorphan worked better than a placebo, though one study did not show that dextromethorphan helped at all. That is not a ringing endorsement for dextromethorphan, but at least there is the possibility that it works. For children, none of these anti-coughing medicines seems to work at all, including codeine and dextromethorphan. Studies of other pediatric cough syrups did not show any benefits for children's coughs or other symptoms.

Another kind of medicine for coughs is an expectorant. An expectorant helps to dissolve or thin your mucus, which may make it easier to cough up that nasty stuff in your lungs. For adults, one type of expectorant called guaifenesin seems to help those who take it four times a day to cough less hard and less often; however, there is no evidence that this type of medicine works for children.

You may have noticed that children do not seem to benefit from any of these medicines. Although over-the-counter cough and cold medicines are frequently used in children, the scientific data suggest that they do not actually work! In six randomized placebo-controlled studies testing the use of cough and cold medicines in children under the age of twelve, the scientists could not find any difference between taking a cough and cold medicine or taking a placebo medicine. No one knows exactly why these medicines do not work for kids, but the science is clear that they do not!

Even worse than not working, these medicines have a higher risk of negative side effects in children, especially in the youngest children. In safety data from the United States Food and Drug Administration (FDA) that report on the use of these medicines over the course of thirty-seven years (1969–2006) for children younger than six, fifty-four children were deemed to have died because of side effects from decongestants and sixty-nine died from side effects from antihistamines. Usually, an overdose of these medicines was responsible for the child's death. Children can actually die from these medicines! Many more children have bad side effects from these medicines that do not kill them, but that require medical treatment. In the United States in 2004–2005, 1,519 children under the age of two had to go to the emergency room for treatment because of negative side effects from over-the-counter cough and cold medicines. These side effects can include serious conditions like abnormal heart rhythms and loss of consciousness. Because of these bad side effects (and also because these medicines don't work!), the FDA has issued more strict advisories cautioning against the use of these medicines in young children, especially for children less than two years old. As pediatricians, we advise you not to give your babies and toddlers these medicines. And talk to your doctor before you administer them to your older children.

In conclusion, no over-the-counter medicines for colds and cough are effective for kids, and many are not effective even for adults. Dextromethorphan and guiafenesin for cough, antihistamine-decongestant combinations for general symptoms, and at least the first dose of nasal decongestants may offer some benefit for adults. For children, none of these medicines offers clear benefits and many have been associated with bad side effects, so they are best avoided altogether.

Croup

Cool mist will help your child's croup

When babies get croup, they have a terrible, barking cough and can get to a point where they have a lot of trouble breathing. Pediatricians will usually recommend that parents put these babies in a humid place, like the bathroom with the shower running, in order to help with the cough and breathing difficulties. Doctors will also sometimes use special plastic tents with humidified air or humidified breathing treatments when croup sends a baby to the hospital. Parents may even start using humidifiers in order to prevent babies from having these problems. If you ask most doctors, they would say that humidified mist will help your child's croup. Doctors have used mist like this since the nineteenth century, when physicians felt that the steam from teapots and hot tubs alleviated croup symptoms.

Pediatricians and parents alike may be surprised to learn that there is no evidence to support using humidified air to treat croup. There have only been a few studies looking at this, but none have shown a benefit. A study from 1978 in Britain showed no improvement when using a saline mist (nebulized saline) for children with croup. Another study, done in Australia in 1984, randomized children with croup to either a normal environment or to an enclosed cot where they were surrounded by cool, humid mist. The children were evaluated throughout twelve hours, and there were no differences between the groups in terms of their clinical conditions, vital signs, and the amount of oxygen in their blood.

Two subsequent randomized, controlled studies done in Canada showed no evidence that humidity improved croup symptoms of children in the emergency department. A study of dogs showed that airway resistance (which is higher than it should be when a child has croup) actually got better with dry air than with moist air. In fact, both cool dry air and hot dry air created lower airway resistance than cool moist air or hot moist air. A meta-analysis that searched for all of the available studies testing humidified air for croup in children, found that the combined studies did not support using humidified air for croup. It just does not work.

However, we shouldn't throw out the baby with the bathwater. If sitting with Mom in a bathroom with the shower going makes both Mom and child calmer, then by all means do it. But maybe we should think twice before we advocate holding that mist tube in front of a screaming, thrashing kid in the emergency department, or placing a baby in a croup tent that separates him from loving care.

Dairy

If you are sick, you should stay away from dairy products (milk makes you phlegmy)

We have tried to debunk this myth before, but even our supporters have trouble believing that milk does not give them a lot more mucus. A pharmacist friend named Sonak, who considers himself a huge fan of medical myth-busting, just cannot believe that milk does not increase his phlegm and congestion when he's sick. "I can feel it!" he insists. He thinks it is one myth where we are wrong. So we'll look at the science again. If milk is going to make you more congested when you are sick, then we would hate to recommend the wrong thing.

Sonak has plenty of supporters on this one. Drinking milk or consuming other dairy products has long been thought to be associated with increased respiratory problems, congestion, or even with asthma. It has been a traditional Chinese medicine tenet to cut down on how much dairy you are taking in if you have too much mucus in your system. A twelfth-century physician, Moses Maimonides, recommended that people with breathing or congestion problems needed to eliminate milk and dairy from their diets. Even Dr. Spock said that children should not have milk when they have colds! Many of today's doctors recommend the exact same thing; in a study of 330 parents, almost 60 percent believed that milk would increase their child's mucus production, and almost a third of them got this information from their doctor.

Scientists have recently developed a hypothesis to help explain how milk might increase mucus production. We thought

Sonak would be interested in this new theory. In the scheme of how allergies usually work, it did not make sense that milk would give you more congestion instead of, for example, giving you a rash or irritating your digestive tract. Scientists found that when milk is broken down by your body one of the chemicals it becomes is beta-casomorphin-7. The reason you might care about beta-casomorphin-7 if you think milk makes you phlegmy is that this chemical stimulates mucus production from certain glands that line the inside of your gut, specifically the colon. The scientists proposed that maybe this same chemical makes the glands inside your respiratory tract produce more mucus too. It is not yet time to say that Sonak is right and we are wrong. There are a number of reasons why we are not yet convinced by the science. First, there is no evidence that this chemical from milk stimulates the glands in your respiratory tract and makes them produce more mucus. Second, even if it is stimulating glands in your gut, there is no evidence that this would have an impact on your respiratory tract. The chemical would need to get to your respiratory tract, and that's a separate set of pipes from your digestive tract. The two only intersect in the back of your throat. If milk is going down the respiratory set of pipes, you have more problems than just mucus—you will choke! For this chemical that is made in your digestive tract to have an effect in your lungs, it would need to be absorbed into the bloodstream in a way that also causes inflammation in your lungs. There is no evidence that this happens.

In contrast to this unproven idea, there are a lot of scientific studies that seem to prove that there is no link between drinking milk and becoming phlegmy. When tested carefully in human beings, there is no evidence that milk or dairy increases your mucus production. In one test of this idea, scientists took 125 volunteers and randomly assigned them to get cow's milk or a soy drink, both of which were flavored with cocoa and peppermint in a way that made it impossible for the volunteers to know which drink they were getting. The scientists asked all of the participants to rank how much of a mucus effect they had after drinking either product and to describe what their symptoms were. When people did not know whether they were getting dairy milk or a soy drink, they could not tell any difference between how the drinks affected them. There was no difference in having a "coating over the mouth," "swallowing a lot," or having "thicker saliva" whether you drank milk or soy. However, if you believed beforehand that milk gave you more mucus, then you reported more of these problems for either of the beverages.

In another great study of this myth, scientists took sixty volunteers and tried to make them sick with the common cold virus by sticking it directly in their nose. Then they carefully recorded the volunteers' breathing symptoms and their milk and dairy intake over the next ten days. Even better, they actually measured the weight of the sick people's snot to see how much mucus they were making! (Take a moment to be glad that you don't have a job measuring people's mucus weight.) Fifty-one of those volunteers got sick, but how much dairy they were taking in did not have any impact on how they felt. Drinking more milk was not associated with any increase in problems with coughing, congestion, or a runny nose, nor did drinking more milk change the weight of their nasal secretions. In other studies that look at adults with asthma, researchers also found that there was no effect on their breathing, coughing, or wheezing from drinking either whole or skim milk. It was the same as drinking water. This was also true in a study looking at patients with eczema and asthma. If they did not have any actual milk allergy, the milk did not do anything to flare up their asthma or their eczema. These are very careful studies, testing this idea in human beings, and showing no impact from milk.

Are we saying that milk causing more mucus is all in your head? Not entirely. People who believe that milk causes more mucus seem to be sensitive to the sensation that milk creates in the mouth. Though milk does not actually increase the amount of mucus your body makes or change how congested you are, you might feel something different in your mouth when you drink it. Experts tell us that milk spreads out in tiny droplets over the saliva in your mouth. The official name for this process is called "droplet flocculation." The feeling of those tiny droplets in your mouth might be mistaken for having more mucus, especially among people who are very sensitive to this sensation. You also might be interested to know that drinking any fluid—water and milk alike—increases the amount of saliva that you have, though studies show neither makes your saliva thicker.

Even if you think something is happening and feel something different, this does not make it real! The studies have showed that people who are "sensitive" to milk's effects can be fooled in the same way by soy drinks. Milk does not make your cold or breathing worse.

Day Care

Kids in day care catch more colds

If you have children or work with them, you know that they are prone to endless runny noses and coughs and sniffles, especially during the winter months. Children average between six and ten colds per year. Since respiratory infections typically last for ten to fourteen days, that is a lot of days out of every month with some sort of cold or respiratory infection. For children in day care, parents often feel like the situation is even worse. Children in day care seem to be sick all the time, and this makes some parents feel especially guilty about leaving their children.

There is some truth to this concern. Attending day care has been associated with more respiratory infections, but it is difficult to know what other factors are coming into play. While several studies have found higher rates of respiratory infections in children attending day care, studies have also found that children are sick more days when they have more siblings and when they come from poorer households.

It is also important to track where in a child's lifespan they get sick. Very large studies show us that children in day care do get sick more often when they first start going, but these infections are less common as time goes on. As the children get older, they have no more infections than those children who are cared for at home, and they seem to have fewer illnesses once they are school-aged. This could be because they have been exposed to more viruses and bugs early on, so their immune system protects them well by the time they are in school. A Danish study looked at more than 135,000 children in Copenhagen, and found that the youngest children attending day care, those under two years old, were at a higher risk of catching colds than children who are cared for at home. In their first six months of going to day care, children younger than two years have much higher rates of getting sick than children who stay home. This is especially true for young children who do not have any other siblings. However, the risk decreases as the children get a bit older.

Parents who are concerned about all of the day care sicknesses need to balance this with what happens when children get sick when they are a bit older. Another study found that children who go to large day care centers when they are in preschool have fewer colds in later years, doing better than their peers in terms of not getting sick and not missing school when they are up to thirteen years old. The day care kids seem to have built up their immunity to common colds and viruses earlier in life, and they benefit from that once school starts, whereas the stay-at-home children start to get exposed to all of those viruses only when they hit school.

Deodorants

Deodorants and antiperspirants cause breast cancer

We've already discussed the fact that there are things you can do to prevent cancer. Some things, though, have nothing to do with cancer at all. Because cancer is scary, it sometimes seems like it doesn't take much to inflame the myth-believing part of our brains to swallow as true a made-up story about cancer.

We can't tell you how many times we have been forwarded e-mails from our friends that breathlessly relate how "studies" have proven that deodorants and antiperspirants cause breast cancer. They claim that "someone" doesn't want you to know the truth. Neither of us has any vested interest in the deodorant and antiperspirant market, and all we want you to know are the facts.

Some people believe that toxins in deodorants and antiperspirants enter the blood and cause cancer. Some people believe that shaving your underarms breaks open the skin and lets these toxins in faster. Some people believe that these toxins collect in the lymph nodes in the breast. None of this has been shown to be true.

Most of the published "studies" are not actual studies, or if they are, they're seriously flawed. For instance, a paper appeared in the *European Journal of Cancer Prevention* in 2001 entitled, "Underarm Cosmetics Are a Cause of Breast Cancer." What many people missed was that this manuscript was published under the heading "Hypothesis" and actually was a thought piece in which the author theorized that maybe deodorants and antiperspirants could be a cause of breast cancer. It wasn't a study, and it didn't actually prove anything. But if you just looked at the title and the journal it appeared in, you'd get a completely different picture.

Another influential study published in 2003 declared, "An earlier age of breast cancer diagnosis is related to more frequent use of antiperspirants/deodorants and underarm shaving." This study found that women who were younger and had breast cancer reported shaving their underarms more and starting to use deodorants and antiperspirants earlier. They therefore concluded that shaving underarms and using antiperspirants was associated with earlier onset of breast cancer. There was one huge flaw, though. Since the study examined no women without breast cancer, it's entirely possible that younger women are simply more likely to shave their underarm hair than older women. But we can't tell since there was no comparison group studied of women without breast cancer.

Or can we? In 2002, a study was published that compared about 1,600 women both with and without breast cancer. In that study, no association could be found between shaving underarms or using deodorants and antiperspirants and breast cancer.

You might wonder why most breast cancer occurs in what is called the upper outer quadrant of the breast, nearest to where deodorants and antiperspirants are applied. Generally speaking, this is because most breast tissue is in the upper outer part of the chest. In fact, the American Cancer Society notes that the proportion of breast cancer that occurs in this area of the breast is equal to the proportion of breast tissue that is in that area.

You might also wonder why your doctor has told you not to use antiperspirants when you're getting a mammogram. That's because the aluminum contained in antiperspirants can interfere with the scan. It has nothing to do with concerns for your health.

Breast cancer is a serious problem with a large impact on the health of women. There are things we can do to help women avoid breast cancer and detect it sooner. But giving up deodorants and antiperspirants will do nothing to prevent it.

Echinacea

I have just the thing for that cold . . . Echinacea

The echinacea flower is widely believed to be an effective remedy for your sniffles and snot. Many people believe that echinacea is an immune stimulator that helps protect your body against getting colds or even fights them off. Unfortunately, there is little scientific evidence in support of echinacea fighting colds.

Studies including as many as 3,000 people have looked at whether echinacea prevents colds and whether it treats upper respiratory tract infections or colds. For neither purpose does echinacea stand up to scrutiny. The results of the studies are difficult to combine into a final set of results because they look at different parts of the plant and they use different methods for their studies. Nonetheless, an overview of the studies suggests that echinacea just does not perform as well as we would like it to.

In 2006, a Cochrane systematic review examined all of the evidence from studies of echinacea. The Cochrane systematic reviews are considered the highest-quality reviews that summarize the science of a particular subject. In sixteen studies of the herb, echinacea did no better than a sugar pill (placebo) for preventing or treating colds. In the best studies, where the volunteers either received a placebo or else received echinacea, the majority of studies did not find any benefit for echinacea in preventing colds. When you look only at the less well done studies, those that did not use placebos, scientists more often find just a suggestion that echinacea helps to prevent colds. When only the lower-quality studies show an effect, we worry that biases and bad science are influencing the outcome. The results from the better-quality studies are more trustworthy. These studies tell us that echinacea does not prevent colds. The summary of the high-quality studies also concludes that echinacea does not work to treat colds or cold symptoms. In an example of one of the well-crafted studies that was published in the *New England Journal of Medicine,* doctors divided 400 volunteers into groups that either took a sugar pill or took echinacea. They found that taking echinacea did not change the severity of a volunteer's cold, nor did it change how the cold progressed.

Some of the studies examining whether echinacea treats colds have found a small improvement in the duration of cold symptoms when echinacea is used for adults. In these, echinacea led to slightly shorter colds in adults, but the results were mixed. For children, echinacea does not improve cold symptoms and can lead to side effects like a bad rash. Once again, when studies show only very small potential benefits, we have to temper our expectations. It is possible that echinacea has a small effect on the duration of the cold, but the effect is not powerful enough to consistently turn up in studies of the herb.

Compilations of studies that were done after the Cochrane review compilation have not provided any more convincing evidence in favor of echinacea. In 2007, a group of researchers claimed that the evidence from fourteen studies suggested that echinacea did shorten cold symptoms by a day or so. Unfortunately, other researchers claimed that those scientists did not combine the studies appropriately and that the results could not be trusted. Another group compiled studies where researchers put the cold virus right into the noses of study participants and then followed up to see if the herb did anything to stop the people with virus in their nose from getting sick.

This is a great way to design studies of whether something works for colds, but echinacea did not work. We know it can be confusing when the science does not agree on a particular topic. In this case, most of the science says that echinacea does not work. And if echinacea does work for helping cold symptoms, the results are not strong enough to produce consistent results. The bottom line is that echinacea does not prevent colds. While echinacea might make your cold linger for a little less time, that is pretty unlikely too.

Eggs

Eggs give you high cholesterol

For decades, eggs have been getting a bad rap. Everyone "knows" you shouldn't eat a lot of eggs, and they all think they know why. The logic goes like this: eggs are high in cholesterol, people who eat a lot of cholesterol in their diet get high levels of cholesterol in their blood, and people with high levels of cholesterol in their blood are more likely to have heart disease. So, if you want to avoid heart disease, don't eat eggs. That was easy.

Let's look at this more closely. The first one is easy to acknowledge. Each egg contains about 212 mg of cholesterol. Of course, that assumes you eat the yolk, since egg whites have no cholesterol whatsoever, but we'll assume you're eating the whole egg. Since the daily recommended allowance for cholesterol is 300 mg, that egg does seem to contain a lot of cholesterol in it. But eggs are also a source of great nutrition. Eggs are a good source of protein. They also contain vitamins, minerals, and unsaturated fats (which your body needs). They also contain choline, lutein, and zeaxanthin, which sound odd but may also help to prevent eye and heart disease. So it's not like eggs are empty cholesterol bombs.

The second leg of the argument is more complicated. Basically, the theory is that if you eat things high in cholesterol (like eggs), you get high cholesterol in your blood or high serum cholesterol. Serum cholesterol is the cholesterol level you (should) get checked at your doctor each year. And there is some truth to the theory. But the link between high dietary cholesterol and high serum cholesterol is not nearly as strong as you think. This theory that diet cholesterol increases serum cholesterol only occurs in hyperresponders. These are people who really respond to dietary cholesterol, and they are a minority. About 70 percent of people are what are known as hyporesponders. These people show no increase in their serum LDL—"bad" cholesterol—after eating three eggs a day for thirty days. For the majority of people, there is not a clear link between eating eggs and having really high bad cholesterol in their blood.

It gets worse (or better depending on your outlook). Good research estimates that even in hyperresponders, for every extra 100 mg of cholesterol in your diet, your serum cholesterol goes up about 2 mg per deciliter. That's not nearly as much as you think. So adding a daily egg to your diet may increase your serum cholesterol by 4 mg/dl. That's not the difference between a heart attack and no heart attack. This is especially true since other research shows that eggs preferentially cause an increase in large LDL molecules, which are less damaging than smaller ones. Additionally, an increase in HDL, or the "good" cholesterol, also occurs.

The final nail in the coffin of this argument comes when you look at studies of heart disease. A large study of male physicians found that eating up to six eggs a week did not increase the risk of heart failure. Eating more than seven eggs a week did. But this was a study of only male physicians. Another study, a bigger and better one looking at 120,000 men and women, showed no difference in the risk of heart attack or stroke over a fourteen-year period if you ate one or more eggs a day compared to eating an average of one egg per week. Eggs just don't seem to lead to heart disease in otherwise healthy people.

We're not advocating that people go right out and eat an unhealthy diet high in cholesterol. But the wholesale avoidance of eggs is an overreaction that has no basis in science. Eggs can be a part of a very healthy diet, and do not deserve the terrible reputation they seem to have developed.

Raw eggs will give you salmonella

Eggs get a bad rap all around. They are blamed for raising your cholesterol, and time and time again we hear about people getting terribly sick with salmonella from eggs. In the 1990s, U.S. government reports suggested that as many as 20 percent of all U.S. chickens were contaminated with salmonella, although later reports dropped that number to as low as 3 percent. Even with the lower numbers, you may worry that eggs are a dangerous food, at least when it comes to food poisoning! Raw eggs, in particular, may inspire panic. The fear of raw eggs is great enough that Rachel worries a little every time she sneaks a lick of the uncooked brownie or cookie batter.

The truth is that eggs, raw or cooked, are not the risky food that you might think. Eggs cause only a tiny percentage—0.5 percent—of all of the illnesses that people in the United States contract from food every year.

But even if it is a small risk, you might still be worried about eggs and salmonella. After all, salmonella are nasty bacteria that can cause bad diarrhea, fever, vomiting, and cramps and can even be fatal in some severe cases. Stories of egg recalls and egg farms being shut down because of salmonella are enough to make any of us scared. And it is true that eggs can be contaminated with salmonella.

Remember, though, that eggs get a bad rap. Despite what you may hear on the news, salmonella does not always come from eggs. It can come from eggs, but up to 85 percent of the cases of people sick with salmonella are unrelated to eggs. Moreover, current estimates are that only 1 in every 30,000 eggs is contaminated by salmonella.

The Centers for Disease Control (CDC) tells us that there are several simple steps to make sure that you do not get ill from any bacteria that might be contaminating your eggs. The first step is to keep your eggs refrigerated. If eggs are refrigerated, salmonella and other bacteria that may be present in or on the eggs should not grow. Second, you should cook the eggs until the yolks are firm and cook foods containing eggs thoroughly. Cooking eggs properly should destroy any salmonella that is present.

This advice about cooking eggs properly makes most of us think that the raw egg is to blame for the salmonella. This is not really true. If salmonella is lurking on the egg, it is actually on the shell of the egg, not inside the yolk or white. Usually, the egg's shell protects the yolk and the egg white against contamination. The problem comes in when the eggshell is cracked open or if there are small cracks in the eggshell; cracking allows the salmonella to infect the rest of the egg. Because of the risk of salmonella coming in from the shell, people are also advised to wash eggs before cracking them open, and to throw out any eggs that have cracks in them. Washing the eggs, plus cooking them thoroughly to kill any salmonella that might have snuck in, should be a good protection against the bacteria.

We are not saying that you should eat raw eggs with wild abandon. Cooked eggs are definitely safer. While there is only a 1 in 30,000 chance that you will be coming across an egg with salmonella on the shell, it is still a risk and one that you can minimize through washing and cooking. Moreover, it always makes sense to use extra caution around people with immune systems that are not as strong, especially children and the elderly. But you should not be afraid of eggs! If you take basic steps to refrigerate, clean, and cook your eggs, they are a healthy protein source.

Exercise

If you stop exercising, your muscles will turn to fat

A aron recently went on an exercise and diet program called P90X. With great zeal, he followed this workout routine and diet for ninety intense days, during which he sculpted his pale, soft body into a much more buff version. And it worked! At the pool, friends admired his newly defined muscles. We have been debunking a lot of health myths, but there are some good health truths to remember. Among the more important is that exercising and building up your muscles are great ways to help your body stay healthy.

Now that Aaron has his bulging P90X muscles, what will happen to them when he stops his crazy workout routine (which he did while writing this book)? Will his muscles soften into pudgy fat? Aaron is great at following diet and exercise plans, but even he might have difficulty finding a way to maintain these muscles.

Aaron can take comfort in one thing, though—it is a myth that muscle will turn into fat when you stop exercising. It is just not true. Fat cells and muscle cells are different things, and one cannot convert into the other. Cells are the smallest functional units in your body, the building blocks of how you are put together as a living creature. You have fat cells, muscle cells, blood cells, bone cells, and so on. These cells do not convert from one kind into another. Muscle cells and fat cells look very different and work in different ways. Muscle cells are mostly a bundle of fibers or filaments that are attached to each other and contract when electricity from the body's nerves come into the cell. Muscle cells are like tiny ropes, powered by small engines and connected together to do the work of pulling your bones around. In contrast, fat cells do not seem like they do very much. Under a microscope, they look like motionless globs. These cells are focused on storing fat and making fat from things like sugar. Fat cells do have jobs; they provide your body with emergency food, they insulate your body, and they help facilitate hormonal activity in your body.

When Aaron stops his P90X program, his muscle cells will not go away. If he stops doing his pull-ups and starts eating food that has a bit more fat in it, he will not have any fewer muscle cells; however, Aaron's muscle cells will get smaller and thinner. He will not develop any more fat cells, but the fat cells that his body has will get bigger and bigger as they store more fat inside them and use less. The muscle and fat cells will not change in number, and the muscle cells will not become fat cells. Instead, the muscle cells will be getting smaller while the fat cells are getting bigger. As the fat cells get bigger, it might look like Aaron's muscles are turning into fat.

There are a few other dimensions to this idea of muscle turning into fat. If a person is really desperate for energy, such as a person who is starving and cannot get enough food, the body can break down some of your muscle fibers to use them for energy. If the muscle fibers are used for energy (by breaking them down through a process called catabolism into the body's sugar source of glucose), and if this happens to such an extent that there is extra sugar left over that the body does not need, then the body will store that sugar as fat. This is pretty rare, as it requires you to need to use parts of your body as an energy source in the place of having food, and yet you need to do this to an extent where you have some leftover to store as fat. The scenario where you let your muscles get small and wasted (from not exercising them) while your fat cells store up more fat (because you are eating more calories than you burn up) is much more common. Interestingly enough, the number of fat cells in your body remains almost constant throughout your life. Some of the fat cells die, and others replace them, but you do not grow brand-new fat cells when you get fat. Instead, your fat cells get bigger and bigger as they store more and more fat.

Eyes

Don't cross your eyes . . . they'll get stuck that way!

You probably remember hearing this one from your mother. When you used to torment your younger sister with gruesome faces, your mother would catch a glimpse of your crossed eyes and scold you, "Don't cross your eyes! They'll get stuck that way!"

This is a case where your mother was just plain wrong (or she was lying to you). There is absolutely no medical or scientific evidence that crossing your eyes will make your eyes stay crossed. Experts in ophthalmology conclude that crossing your eyes voluntarily is absolutely not going to hurt them permanently.

Even though your mother was wrong about the dangers of your silly faces, eye-crossing can be a problem for other reasons. If someone has crossed eyes without trying to cross them, this is a medical condition that merits further investigation. Two to 4 percent of the population has strabismus, in which one or both eyes are not aligned properly and may look crossed. However, you do not develop strabismus as a result of crossing your eyes too often or for too long. Most of the time, babies are born with it. When strabismus or this improper alignment develops later in life, it is usually caused by serious infections or problems in the head such as certain types of brain tumors. If you notice that your child's eyes seem to be crossed or aligned abnormally, you should definitely talk to your doctor about your concerns, but the child's penchant for making silly faces should not be blamed.

The eye is a very complex thing. Eye movements are con-trolled by three pairs of muscles that work in concert. One mus-cle in the pair relaxes and one muscle contracts in order to move the eye in a particular way. Crossing the eyes, or bringing both eyes closer to the nose, is actually the normal movement of the eyes when you are focusing on something very close to your face. When you cross your eyes, you are just mimicking or exaggerat-ing that natural movement. When there are problems in how the eye is moving, doctors need to evaluate which of the muscles in a pair are having difficulty.

We're not saying that crossing your eyes for a long time is the best thing for the muscles of your eyes. It can cause strain in these muscles, which may result in a temporary pain or even in some eye spasms and blurring of your vision. Thankfully, these effects are temporary; when you stop crossing your eyes, the muscles have a chance to rest and the pain or spasms should subside. Your eyes will not be stuck in the crossed position. In the same way, if you use the muscles in your arm to curl a heavy weight, your bi-ceps might feel tired, sore, and even somewhat crampy, but your arm will not be stuck in the curled position. The muscles just need a break to return to feeling normal.

Rubbing your eyes is bad for you—TRUE

With the exception of busting the myth on reading in the dark, no myth was going to be as satisfying to throw in our mothers' faces as this one. Aaron especially was looking forward to rubbing his eyes in abandon and gleefully ignoring his mother's pleas to stop.

We are heartbroken to report that we won't have that pleasure.

The medical literature is shockingly full of bad things that happen to people who rub their eyes too much. One woman is described as having recurrent keratoconus (a really bad eye dis-ease) because of too much vigorous rubbing of her eyes. Another patient was shown to develop migraine headaches because of eye-rubbing.

Similar studies of animals don't help our cause either. One study of rats showed that five minutes of eye-rubbing significantly disrupted the cells lining the conjunctivae (the pink part of eyelids) and caused changes to the cells.

Reviews of the medical literature report that eye-rubbing can double the pressure inside your eyes. If you close your eyes tightly and rub hard, you can increase the pressure in your eyes tenfold. Researchers conclude that eye-rubbing can lead to bad things in individuals susceptible to certain disorders of the eye.

When there is no evidence that something is bad, we are more than happy to tell you. But here is a case where such evidence does seem to exist. The overall risks may be low, but they are real. Your mom was right. Don't rub your eyes.

Fever

Feed a cold, starve a fever

There's a great Calvin and Hobbes cartoon where the little boy is staring at a cow, particularly its udder. And he remarks that you have to wonder who looked at that and thought, whatever comes out of that, I'm going to drink it.

Where do some of these things come from?

We ask because eating is pretty simple when you come down to it. If you're hungry, eat. If you're not, don't. Humans (and animals) have been doing it for years. And there are no animals out there giving each other instructions on how to eat if they're sick. We imagine if they're hungry, they eat, and if they aren't hungry, they don't.

Anyway, at some point, we humans decided we knew better. And we started dispensing this gem. Some believe the origins of this date back to the 1500s, when John Withals, who wrote dictionaries, penned, "Fasting is a great remedie of feuer." Others have hypothesized that eating generates heat, which would be bad in a fever (when you're hot), but good when you're cold. Unfortunately, when you have a cold, you're not necessarily cold in temperature, but logic never stopped any of these myths before.

This is an amazing thing about some of these myths. Even though there is no good reason to believe the idea at face value and no reason to think that the rest of the animal world has been suffering because they lacked such wisdom, we believe in the idea so strongly that we try to prove it true.

This has led to a number of studies trying to see if eating or not eating affects the immune system. A study of six (yes, only six) healthy men found that nutritional status did change the balance of T helper 1 (Th1)–Th2 cells. Moreover, eating resulted in increased levels of gamma interferon, while food deprivation increased interleukin-4 release. In this small study, eating did result in some small changes in the cells of the immune system.

This study did not look at people who had colds or fevers, it did not test any hard outcomes such as whether people get better or not, and, we reiterate, it was a study of just six healthy males. To counter it, we would offer hundreds of millions of years of evolution of animals eating when they are hungry and not eating when they are not.

We suspect that many people will continue to believe this myth. In fact, if you search the literature thoroughly—and we did—you will find a number of articles that continue to offer hypotheses for why this advice is sound. It's important to note, though, that nearly all of these articles state right up front that they are guesses. They aren't studies proving this myth is true. They are attempts to imagine scenarios as to why it might be true.

But that's not research. That's not evidence. There are no studies whatsoever showing that feeding a cold or starving a fever does any more good than harm. The body continues to need fluids when it is sick, but food it can do without for short periods of time. So we say, when you are sick, you should eat when you're hungry! If you're not hungry, wait until you are. Common sense.

If your temperature hits 104, you are going to have brain damage

Of all the symptoms of illness, none seems to inspire panic and concern more than a fever. Parents especially seem madly concerned with the temperature of their children. While some are willing to ignore all sorts of complaints and issues, almost no parent will ignore a bump in temperature.

This problem with fixating on the temperature as a number is that it misses the holistic picture of health and illness. It also causes plenty of needless worry as mothers and fathers watch over their children with rising temperatures, as if by will they could cool them.

In general, fever is just one more symptom of being sick. Like a cough, it is part of the body's armament for fighting infection, not some evil harm dreamed up by devilish germs. The body is usually kept in the range of 98–99 degrees; the idea that all humans exist at 98.6 degrees at all times is actually a myth. In fact, the normal temperature of babies and small children can vary from 97 to 100 degrees depending on the time of day, whether they have eaten recently, or what activities they are engaging in. Anything below 100.4 degrees Fahrenheit is usually not acknowledged as a fever by medical personnel.

The hypothalamus is part of your brain that works (among other things) as your body's thermostat. Fever is caused when the hypothalamus resets your body's temperature. When you are infected with bacteria or viruses, your white blood cells will release a compound called interleukin-1, which alerts the hypothalamus to raise the temperature in your body. Those chills you feel? That shivering that concerns so many of you? Those are part of the way the body gets the job done to fight infections. Raising the temperature is thought to help weaken the germs' capabilities and bring about their death.

Antipyretics, or drugs that help bring down a fever, do so by lowering the hypothalamus's thermostat. The usual drugs to lower fevers are acetaminophen (Tylenol) and ibuprofen. And there is usually nothing wrong with giving these drugs to someone who has a fever. If you have a young baby, you should always talk to a doctor before giving them medicines, but in general, no studies have shown that using medicines to lower your temperature back toward normal will hinder your body's immune system.

Now, back to the numbers. Generally, adults feel worse when they have fevers than do children. An adult with a fever of 104 will usually feel very ill, but 104 is still not high enough to cause concern about potential brain damage. It is highly unlikely that brain damage will occur until your temperature goes over 107.5 for an adult and 106.5 for a child.

That almost never happens. That's because your hypothalamus is in control of your body's temperature. It's not that the infection is driving your temperature up and your body is fighting it. Your body is driving the temperature up on purpose, on its own. And the temperature is not going to be set that high by the hypothalamus. In order to hit temperatures that high, usually something else has to be seriously wrong. If you're seriously dehydrated, for example, your body may not be able to cool itself. If you wrap a child in tons of blankets, then the child also could be in danger because they would not have the ability to cool themselves adequately.

This brings us to some things you should *not* do in an attempt to bring down fever:

Do not try to cool a child with rubbing alcohol. Children can actually absorb the alcohol through their skin, and that is bad.

Do not try to cool a person down with ice water; that's counterproductive.

Do not even try to cool them down with lukewarm water until some time after you've given them antipyretics. If you try and cool them before the hypothalamus has reset itself, you will just be fighting the body as it works in the opposite direction to get the temperature back up.

People do worry that if a temperature goes too high that they might have a seizure. It is true that febrile seizures do occur, but most people now believe that the actual value of the temperature has little to do with seizing. The vast majority of febrile seizures occur at temperatures below 104.

Most important, don't become so fixated on the temperature that you forget to look at the whole picture. Some children with a temperature of 104 can look amazingly well and just have a mild illness. Others can have a temperature of 102 and be seriously ill. Don't overemphasize the fever. It's just one more symptom, and it's very unlikely to cause harm.

Flu

The flu is just a bad cold

We are big fans of flu shots. If you want to debate about whether the flu shot might give you the flu, head to the chapter on vaccines after we try to convince you why you should get a flu shot. One of the arguments we hear most often by people who don't want to get immunized is that the flu just isn't a big deal; it's just a bad cold.

Well, look, there are a number of things the flu and a cold have in common. They both involve the respiratory system and can both include a cough and a runny or stuffy nose. And, of course, they both make you feel sick. But that's where the similarities end.

Colds are caused by a variety of viruses, mostly rhinoviruses (30 to 50 percent) and coronaviruses (10 to 15 percent). The flu, on the other hand, is caused only by the influenza virus. Colds are defined as a short and mild illness first characterized by headache, sneezing, chills, and sore throat; later on you can get a runny or stuffed nose, cough, and feel ill. Usually, things move fast, and colds are at their worst two to three days after infection. Most people feel better in a week to ten days after the cold starts, but some symptoms can last for weeks. Very few people with colds develop fevers. Influenza, on the other hand, feels more like getting hit by a truck. Influenza comes on fast with more symptoms like fever, cough, sore throat, headaches, muscle pains, stuffy nose, weakness, and even a loss of appetite. You are likely to feel much worse with the flu. A lot of people think of the flu or influenza as a stomach flu. While you might have a loss of your appetite or an upset stomach, the main effect from influenza is to make you achy, weak, and tired, with a bad cough, fever, and congestion.

Colds rarely do more than annoy us and slow us down. We don't mean to minimize how bad you feel when you're sick with a cold, but you can be pretty sure as to how bad it will get— after a while, you probably experience the same symptoms time and again. Flu, on the other hand, can kill. In fact, the flu kills up to 500,000 people around the world every year. The number of people who die from colds is almost zero.

While there is no cure for the cold, there actually are antiviral medications that can help the flu go away faster. In order for these medications to work, you need to start taking them in the first day or two after you get the flu. It is therefore important to talk to your doctor as soon as possible after you feel sick in flu season. Once those first few days have passed, the medications will no longer do you any good. Although it is difficult to tell a cold from the flu, the best predictors are cough and fever; having both of these symptoms has a positive predictive value of 80 percent in differentiating flu from a cold. This means that if you have a cough and a fever during the flu season, there is a very good chance you have the flu instead of a cough, so talk to your doctor about getting antiviral medicines for the flu.

Most important—there is a vaccine for the flu. The flu shot works! It prevents illness and saves lives. Not to beat a dead horse, but if your physician recommends that you get a shot, you really should get one. The CDC currently recommends the flu shot for many people. You should get the flu shot if you are at high risk for having complications from the flu. You may not think this includes you, but if you are a child six months to five years old, a pregnant woman, an adult fifty years and older, someone with a chronic medical condition (including asthma), or someone who lives in a nursing home or long-term-care facility, then you should get a flu shot every year. If you live with any of the people on that list, if you live with a child who is less than six months old (since they are too young to get the flu shot), or if you are a health care worker, then you should also get a flu shot every year. This list covers most of us. Get a flu shot! Of course, you should still wash your hands and try to stay away from close contact with sick people to avoid both colds and the flu, but the flu shot may save your life or the life of someone close to you by protecting you against the flu.

Garlic

I have just the thing for that cold . . . Garlic

Taking garlic to prevent or treat colds requires some serious trade-offs. Is it better to smell terrible and be accused of excessive paranoia about avoiding vampires or to have the occasional cough and cold? The average adult has two to four colds a year. Will garlic stave off those days lost to sniffling and suffering?

In a comprehensive review of scientific trials of garlic, only one of the five studies identified was considered to be of good enough quality to give us any definitive answers about garlic. Remember, we need to use high-quality research to determine whether the results are trustworthy. In the one good study of garlic, 146 volunteers were randomly assigned to take a garlic supplement every day for twelve weeks or to take a placebo pill. Interestingly enough, the volunteers who were taking garlic had significantly fewer colds than the volunteers who were taking the placebo. The garlic group also had fewer days of illness overall, but the number of days it took for people to recover from their illnesses was the same for both groups. Garlic just might work! Of course, those taking garlic did have some side effects; they reported more rashes and, not surprisingly, having a bad odor. Hmm. It really does come down to bad smell versus fewer colds.

Because this is just one study, the verdict on garlic is still out. This is not a lot of evidence as to whether garlic really does prevent or treat colds. While this one relatively small study suggests that garlic might prevent your getting colds, this needs to be studied again and again, and in more people, in order to determine if garlic really works.

There may be another important consideration to take into account when deciding whether you want to start taking garlic. While we cannot find any studies to prove or disprove this, it seems likely that reeking like garlic might decrease your chances of getting lucky. That's right—people may not want to sleep with someone who stinks. This just might outweigh the benefits of the garlic because not having sex could make you more vulnerable to colds. In a study that closely examined the immune systems of men who had to spend periods of time either masturbating or not masturbating, scientists found that sexual arousal and orgasms increased the number of certain immune cells. The natural killer cells, which are an important part of your body's immune system, came out to the bloodstream when the volunteers were aroused or having orgasms. Getting lucky might improve the function of your immune system!

Garlic may help to prevent or shorten colds, but we would advise careful consideration of the pros and cons while we wait for more data about how well garlic works. If you have a partner with a poor sense of smell, you may want to go ahead and grab some garlic.

Green Snot

If you have green snot, you need an antibiotic

We've attempted to cover this one before, but it's one of those pervasive myths that we just keep having to dispel. Plus, many of you (even the doctors among you) are convinced that the color of snot is the key to knowing just how sick you are. And you're probably convinced that green is the worst color, the one that means infection, and that requires an antibiotic.

Let's start with some basic facts. What makes snot turn green? You might think that working with snot would be so disgusting that no one would ever do it. You'd be wrong.

When you have an infection, the body sends off neutrophils—a type of white blood cell—to fight the infection. So if you have an infection in your nose, it's likely there are more neutrophils present in your nasal passages than usual. These cells work by (for lack of a better description) eating the germs that make you sick. Once they have swallowed or engulfed the germs, the special white blood cells keep the germs in what serves as their "stomachs," and they digest them. One of the enzymes that the white blood cells use most often to digest the invader germs is called myeloperoxidase, and myeloperoxidase has a fair amount of iron in it. (This is important as we continue with the germ-eating story.)

Once the neutrophils get full of digested germs, they burst. The iron in the myeloperoxidase gets mixed into the surrounding stuff in your nose. And when you mix iron into that stuff, guess what color your snot turns? Green.

Notice we said nothing about bacteria here. That's because this works exactly the same for viruses or bacteria. It doesn't matter which of the offending germs are in your nose. Whether bacteria or viruses have invaded doesn't affect the iron in the myeloperoxidase in the neutrophils, and that is what makes your snot green. So you may have green snot with a bacterial infection, but it also may not be bacterial. The green does not tell you if it's a bacterial infection. And only bacterial infections need antibiotics.

This hasn't stopped the battle from being waged, however. Even though this issue has been around for a long time, doctors still vehemently disagree as to whether antibiotics have any effect for conditions with green snot. A lot of doctors, perhaps most doctors, are much more likely to give you an antibiotic if you tell them your snot is green. But even the authors of a study finding a small link between antibiotic use and feeling better say that you shouldn't use antibiotics routinely for green snot. There may have been people with sinusitis in that study, and some of them included people with green snot for almost a month. It's a hotly debated piece.

The bottom line is that you can tell almost nothing about the bug infecting you from the fact that you have green snot. Antibiotics will do nothing for you if you have a viral infection. And many studies confirm that antibiotics are associated with side effects. If an antibiotic is not going to help you and might cause a bad side effect, then you want to avoid using one. If you are sick, you should talk with your doctor about whether treating your infection with antibiotics might cause more good than harm, but do not let the greenness of your snot sway the decision.

G-spot

Women do not have a G-spot

You might be surprised to know just how much controversy exists among sex researchers and gynecologists as to whether women have a G-spot. G-spot is a term used to describe an especially sensitive area that supposedly exists in a woman's vagina. This erogenous zone is supposed to be an area that can be stimulated to lead to pleasurable feelings or even orgasms in women for whom the G-spot can be identified. Among those who say that this spot exists, they suggest it is located on the front wall of the vagina, about halfway between the pubic bone and the cervix. The G-spot is often cited as being a source of "internal" or "vaginal" orgasms for a woman, as opposed to the clitoris, which can be stimulated for more of an "external" orgasm.

The G-spot was named after Dr. Ernst Gräfenberg, a German obstetrician and gynecologist, who described a sensitive female area back in the 1950s. Three researchers, Drs. John Perry and Beverly Whipple, and Alice Kahn Ladas, Ed. D., dubbed this area the G-spot in his honor in their 1982 book called *The G Spot: And Other Discoveries About Human Sexuality*. What they described was really more of an area than a spot, an area on the front wall of the vagina where a number of anatomical structures tend to come together—blood vessels, glands and ducts on either side of the urethra, nerve endings, the vagina wall, and the neck of the bladder. In their study, 400 women were examined, and the G-spot was identified in each one. Histologic studies, ones that look at the types of cells or human tissues, seem to support the existence of this area in terms of the various components coming together in one area. However, they also suggest that the composition of this area is somewhat different from one woman to another, which may be why it seems like some women do not have a G-spot or do not experience pleasure when this area is stimulated. Contrary to popular belief, the G-spot does not have a lot more nerve endings. In a study that took 110 biopsies from twenty-one women, they did not find a particular area in this region with lots and lots of nerves. While this small study could have just missed the spot, it also supports the idea that the G-spot is not just a bunch of nerves, but a collection of other structures.

This all sounds fairly straightforward. Surely scientists can tell if a body part exists or not, right? You might be surprised. A number of them doubt whether the G-spot exists at all. However, the science disproving the G-spot is not particularly strong. One argument against the G-spot is that some scans, such as an MRI, have not revealed an obvious structure. The problem with these studies is that they are generally very small. Scientists have argued based on one scan of one woman in whom they did not see a structure that they would call a G-spot. One scan of one woman does not mean that there is not a particularly sensitive area present. Other arguments against the G-spot suggest that there is not a particular anatomical spot, but that the entire area is quite sensitive or that the G-spot might be "in women's heads." If you think that stimulating a particular area is going to feel good, then it will feel good, argue these detractors. The problem with this line of thinking is that it could go either way for the G-spot. Certainly, the brain is an important sexual organ. If you think something will be exciting or you think something will feel good or you want someone to touch you, that should make that aspect of sex more enjoyable! This does not mean that there is no sensitive area in the vagina; it just means that the psychology of sex might be the most important thing overall. Researchers both for and against the G-spot agree with that idea.

Another recent study claimed to disprove the existence of the G-spot based on a study in 1,800 twins. Just over half of the women believed they had a G-spot, but the twins of these women were no more likely to think that they had a G-spot. The lack of a twin connection made the study authors conclude that this was evidence against an anatomical G-spot. While twins should be more likely to have the same anatomical structures, it is also possible that their sexual experiences are different enough that they do not consider themselves sensitive in the same areas. As the G-spot expert Dr. Whipple suggests, the biggest problem with this study is that twins usually do not have the same sexual partner! With different people, different emotions, and different scenarios, the experience of sexuality among the twins might be different enough to color whether they think they have this sensitive area.

After reviewing the studies of the G-spot, it is clear that experts are divided and that the science is not rigorous enough to give us a clear answer. On balance of these data, we are going to come down in favor of the existence of the G-spot. (We're trying to be very scientific, but have to admit that there are likely some nonscientific reasons biasing this conclusion. We'll spare you the specifics . . .) Reasonable examinations have supported the existence of the G-spot, and no convincing science currently disproves these findings. One of the most important factors here is how important the brain is to the experience of sexuality. The reason to celebrate the G-spot is not because women should be pressured to find if they have such an area and to have it stimulated. Instead, it should refocus us to know more about the parts of the body that can be involved in pleasurable experiences. It is also clear that more research needs to be done related to women's sexuality, even in the basics of the anatomy of the vagina.

Hair Dye

Dyeing your hair will give your baby birth defects

According to the American Cancer Society, about 70 percent of adult women use hair dye. So it only stands to reason that a significant number of pregnant women are going to be faced with the fact that they would be due for a reapplication while they're pregnant. As with everything else in pregnancy, the question comes up as to what potential harm dyeing your hair might do to the fetus.

Many people, and many organizations, will tell you that dyeing your hair is dangerous for your baby. Hair dyes use harsh chemicals. Chemicals are absorbed through your head (or hands if you touch the stuff) and then seep into your blood, get carried to your unborn baby, and cause horrific problems like birth defects or cancer. (Right?)

You wouldn't be crazy for thinking that hair dye could be bad for unborn babies. A widely publicized study was published in 2005, in the aptly named journal *Cancer Causes and Control*, which described a link between the use of maternal hair dye and the subsequent risk of neuroblastoma, a type of cancer, in their children.

Here's the thing. That was a case-control study, and as we have discussed, that type of study is really susceptible to recall bias, where people remember things differently because they have a problem. Here's how the study went. They telephoned over 500 mothers who had children with neuroblastoma. They asked the mothers about potential risk factors for cancer, including a lot of questions about hair dye use. Then they randomly called a similar number of people whose children did not have neuroblastoma and asked them the same question. They found that 23 percent of case mothers reported hair dye use, compared to 16 percent of control mothers. It is well known that people whose children have the disease (cases) are more likely to report stuff that might have caused the disease than people whose children don't have the disease (controls). That's recall bias. Moreover, you have to remember that this study does not prove that hair dye causes neuroblastoma; at best, it can show an association. The association was not even particularly strong.

The authors do note these limitations of the study, and ended the paper by calling for more research. There have been a number of studies of hair dye in pregnant animals. A study of twelve rabbits and twenty cats given hair dye many times during a pregnancy could find no effects in their offspring. Another study of five different hair dyes given to rats found no effects. This study also used a control of megadoses of vitamin A to prove that rats exposed to some compounds would have abnormal fetuses (they did). There are others, showing similar results.

Still, for some of you, any risk is too much. We understand that. But consider that you likely engage in many activities each day that are of higher risk to your baby than the theoretical and unproven one of dyeing your hair. For example, your risk of being in a car accident that would harm you and the baby is probably much higher than the risk from dyeing your hair. Talk with your doctor, and make your own decision. We know that dyeing hair is very important to some women (no names mentioned), and they should know there really is no evidence proving that dyeing their hair will cause cancer in their children.

Handshakes

Don't shake hands if you want to stay healthy

How many times do we mention the importance of hand washing in this book? Probably a hundred times. All the studies and experts tell us that hand washing is one of the best ways to avoid getting sick. We pick up all kinds of germs on our hands—whether from shaking hands with someone who has been coughing and sneezing their infectious snot all over their palms or by touching contaminated door handles, phones, or faucets. If it is so very important to keep our hands clean, it makes sense that the best course of action might be to avoid any hand-shaking altogether. When the H1N1 influenza, or swine flu, was rapidly spreading around the world, the United States vice president suggested that people should avoid hand-shaking. Many people were left wondering whether they needed to risk offending others by refusing to shake hands.

Hand-shaking is an important tradition in many cultures. In the United States, hand-shaking is particularly important for introductions, making agreements, and bidding farewell. Politicians use hand-shaking to win confidence, approval, and votes. In Kenya, where Rachel works for half of the year, hand-shaking is an expected greeting whenever you meet someone. In fact, a person is expected to shake hands with everyone in the room they enter. Even very young children in Kenya shake hands when they greet adults. Giving up hand-shaking seems like a difficult proposition. Without a handshake, we may feel isolated, missing human contact, or slighted. It may be difficult to know whether you have really reached an agreement if you cannot shake on it. And if you refuse an offered hand, people might think you rude or insulting. But we know that you really do not want to get sick either.

It is absolutely true that you could catch a cold or the flu by shaking someone's hand. Cold sufferers often get mucus or snot on their hands when they cough and sneeze. If you shake their hand and then touch your own mouth or nose, you could get sick too. Even though this is a real risk, there is a simple way that you can break this cycle. Wash your hands! If you wash your hands before you touch your own mouth or nose, you can easily protect yourself from those germs. An alcohol-based hand sanitizer works very well to clean off your hands if you cannot get to a sink and soap easily. In fact, the alcohol hand rubs work better than soap and water in many studies of hand-washing. You can also train yourself to avoid touching your eyes, nose, or mouth with your hands if you have not had a chance to wash your hands. Keep your hands away from your face unless you know they are clean.

It is also important to remember that many other infections are not passed through hand-shaking. As we talked about in some of the previous chapters, a lot of serious infections are actually not very contagious. You can be very close to most sick people without getting sick yourself, and hand-shaking will not pass most serious infections. Moreover, remember the odds; not everyone is sick! In fact, the majority of the people you meet every day are healthy. While you may meet more infected people during the cold and flu seasons, and while it is not a bad idea to wash your hands regularly (or use hand sanitizer) no matter whose hands you are shaking, most people's hands are not going to make you sick.

Doctors do a lot of hand-shaking, and they do a lot of hand-shaking with very sick people. In Rachel's work, she shakes hands with HIV-infected patients all the time. HIV is not passed through hand-shaking, nor are most other serious diseases. As pediatricians, we see countless children with coughs and colds. While these common infections *can* be passed through hand-shaking, even doctors in constant contact with sick people can avoid getting sick most of the time by washing their hands regularly and not touching their mouths or noses very often. The risks of hand-shaking are very small in contrast to the benefits of hand-shaking for greeting each other, for making emotional and business connections, and for affirming our human connections.

Homes

You shouldn't enter the home of someone who is sick

Many common illnesses, from diarrhea to colds, can be spread inside the house of someone sick. Some of these illnesses are spread either by direct contact with secretions (the gross stuff— snot, phlegm, spit, poop) or by breathing in tiny drops of secretions that have been sneezed or coughed into the air. If a person is sick with a viral or bacterial infection that is spread by their secretions, and if you touch something in the house that has those secretions on it, then you might get sick. For example, doorknobs, dirty tissues, or toys that a sick baby has slobbered on could be contaminated and may pass on infections if you touch those things and then put your hands in your mouth. While germs could be aerosolized or present in the air in tiny liquid droplets, this is more of a risk if you are very close to the infected person. However, as the chapter on breathing the same air as a sick person suggests, it is possible for you to catch a bug from the air in the same house as a sick person. The air within residential houses is typically exchanged for outside air less frequently than the air in office buildings. Although this could allow the germs to hang around in the air, you should remember that the average house has far fewer people potentially sending their germs into that air than the average office building.

So, there is a risk, but it is not a huge risk. Many of these germs, whether bacteria or viruses, do not live for very long once they are outside the body. And for many of them, the greatest risk is when you are very close to the sick person, or when the sick person's secretions are freshly coughed or sneezed or slobbered onto things. You have to get a certain number of the germs into your body before they have a good chance at making you sick. Even if you touch or breathe in something contaminated, there may not be enough living germs on that thing to make you sick.

Some of the viruses that cause diarrhea, such as rotavirus, are among the most difficult to escape in a house. In studies, rotaviruses have been able to survive for days to weeks on surfaces around the house, and ingestion of as few as ten rotavirus particles can cause infection. If someone in the house has rotavirus, you should probably try to stay away!

Despite the possibility of getting infected, it is important to remember the big picture. Not all infections are spread through the air or through secretions or body fluids; some would require you to directly touch the infected area on the person. And, of course, some illnesses are not contagious at all. Furthermore, even for infections that are spread through the air or through contact with infected secretions, you still may not get infected even if you are in the same house.

How can you escape infection? First of all, good hand-washing (and not sucking on your fingers or picking your nose with dirty hands) can help you to avoid getting infected from even the most infected secretions that may be around the house. Second, a quick visit is unlikely to hurt you. In a study where sick volunteers spent time living in small quarters with healthy volunteers, it took a long time before anyone passed on infections. Even though the sick people and the volunteers were playing board, card, and video games in close contact with each other throughout the study, it took an average of 200 hours of exposure to the sick people in order for the healthy volunteers to get infected themselves. It is also important to remember that the risk of getting infected in public places with a lot of people is higher than the risk you face with a limited number of people over a short time.

Going into a house with one or two sick people may be less of a risk than being on a subway or bus with a whole bunch of people.

Beyond hand-washing, the Centers for Disease Control and Prevention offers some suggestions for further decreasing the risk of spreading illnesses like influenza within the house. The CDC suggests that linens, dishes, and utensils used by those who are sick do not need to be cleaned separately, but they do caution against sharing these items unless they have been washed first. The CDC even gives laundry advice; they recommend washing towels and bedsheets with regular laundry soap and tumbling them dry on a hot setting. They also suggest that you should not hold laundry against your body and that you should wash your hands after you handle dirty laundry. It is considered safe to wash the sick person's eating utensils in either a dishwasher or by hand with water and soap.

You should also know that people are generally contagious before they have any symptoms from their infections—before they even know they are sick. This seems like a depressing piece of news, but we would argue that you never really know when someone might be getting sick, and so the practical thing is to avoid wasting time being concerned about who may or may not infect you. Instead, practice the basic precautions to avoid infections or illness. Wash your hands!

Honey

I have just the thing for that cold . . .
Honey and Vinegar

Rachel's hair stylist, Jeff, swears that a mixture of hot vinegar and honey will cure any cold or soothe any sore throat. Once, Rachel had the misfortune of going to get her hair cut when she had entirely lost her voice due to a bad cold. While she sat captive in the styling chair, Jeff whipped up a mixture of his hot vinegar and honey cold remedy, and Rachel was strongly encouraged to drink the noxious mixture. Willing to try almost anything once, Rachel forced down the concoction (with only a little gagging) and was grateful that her sense of taste was dulled by her cold. It tasted terrible, and she was left wondering how much it helped.

Jeff is not the only one to recommend honey for a cold or cough. The World Health Organization (WHO) suggests that honey may be a useful treatment for children with colds because it might soothe the throat and provide some cough relief. However, these 2001 guidelines from the WHO recognized that there was no scientific evidence to support that honey actually worked.

Honey might be helpful for a cough or cold for several reasons. Honey is a demulcent, a substance that forms a film or coating over your throat. It is common for cough medicines to contain something that forms this kind of film in your throat because it is thought to be soothing, potentially relieving minor pain and inflammation or irritation of your throat. Honey has also been found to have some antioxidant properties and to stimulate the release of cytokines, chemicals that can cause inflammation but also help your body fight infections.

One good study has been done to look at how honey impacts nighttime coughing and the ability to sleep for coughing children with colds. This study compared honey to a common cough medicine (dextromethorphan), which was flavored and mixed up to look, taste, smell, and feel like honey. As we have mentioned before, studies have shown that dextromethorphan does not help children's coughs. This was also an important comparison because the parents, children, and investigators were blinded to what the children were receiving; they did not know if they were getting real honey or fake honey. The children were also compared to a group of coughing children who did not receive honey or dextromethorphan. This was a well-designed study. Depending on their age, children received one half to two teaspoons of buckwheat honey or fake honey or no treatment at all before they were supposed to go to bed. In the end, the parents of the children who had honey reported less coughing and fewer symptoms of their colds compared to children who received no treatment. The fake honey was not better than receiving no treatment for any of the outcomes. However, comparing the honey directly with the fake treatment did not show any significant differences. The summary of this study is that, when you compare honey, fake honey (regular dextromethorphan cough medicine), and no treatment, parents rate the honey as the best to help get rid of their children's nighttime coughs and help the child and parent sleep. It may not work much better than a fake honey, and it may not help for many other cold symptoms, but honey does seem to help with children's coughs.

Clearly, honey ought to be studied a bit more, but honey may be worth a try when you or your child are coughing and hacking and not sleeping. The one caution is that honey should not be given to children who are under the age of one. There is a small but real risk that infants can get botulism from honey. Botulism is a rare disease that causes paralysis and leads to death if it is not treated. Eating honey in the first year of life has been shown to be a risk factor for infants to develop this serious condition. If your child is older, you should feel free to give honey a chance to help with that cold.

Jeff may have been on the right track about the honey, but the foul vinegar in his cold remedy concoction is a different story. Jeff is in good company with the idea of using vinegar for colds; back around 400 B.C., Hippocrates prescribed vinegar for curing persistent coughs. Many advocates of home remedies suggest that honey and apple cider vinegar is a natural cough remedy. While vinegar can help as an antibacterial agent to clean counters or tiles, there is absolutely no evidence that vinegar helps with coughs or cold symptoms. What is good for the bathroom floor is not necessarily good for your throat. There is no evidence that vinegar helps clinically with coughs or other infections. A lack of evidence is just that—a lack. It is possible that someone could still prove that vinegar and honey works for colds, but there is no reason to believe that it will.

The next time Rachel gets a haircut, she may have to be extra careful to emphasize how great honey can be for coughs. After all, it is never good to offend someone wielding a sharp scissors near your hair (or any other part of your body). She will just keep in mind the limitations to honey's benefits and the good reasons for avoiding terrible-tasting vinegar.

Eating local honey will prevent allergies

Allergies can be debilitating. They can make you feel terrible, and they can interfere with your quality of life. Moreover, many of the medications for allergies, which are all aimed at interfering with how your immune system responds to allergens, can make you feel sleepy. So it's no wonder that people are looking for other options to fight allergies.

That's where honey comes in. There is a theory that honey, made by bees, could be a vaccine for allergies.

Let's back up a step and talk about vaccines first, so you can understand the rationale for why this might work. Vaccines work by giving our body a "taste" of a dangerous infection. Maybe it's something that looks an awful lot like a dangerous bug. Maybe it's a virus that has been inactivated or killed. Either way, the body reacts by creating antibodies to what is in the vaccine so that later, when the body comes into contact with the actual pathogen (the real and dangerous germ), those antibodies are primed and ready to kill the virus or bacterium.

The theory with local honey is that it contains the same pollen that may be causing your allergies, but in much smaller amounts. Therefore, your body gets practice, much like it would with a vaccine, to get ready to fight off the allergen. Later, when you are exposed to the actual pollen, your body is ready to go and your allergies will disappear.

No. It doesn't work.

First of all, many people remove the "local" from the chapter's title and just think that store-bought honey prevents allergies. That doesn't even make sense. Store-bought honey wouldn't contain the local pollens needed to make this possible. And most store-bought honey is sterilized before being packaged so it might not even contain the bad stuff you would need to induce a response.

Even if you get local honey, there are a few problems with this. First of all, the honey wouldn't contain inactivated pollen. It would contain actual pollen, which could induce an allergic reaction. You could make the same argument that just by staying indoors, you would be exposed to small amounts of allergens from outside and get the same effectiveness. That doesn't happen. On the other hand, experts tell us that swallowing some things we are allergic to sometimes helps our immune system react more tolerably to those things that cause our allergies. Other experts have wondered if honey might contain some sort of antihistamine, acting like the medicines that treat allergies. Neither seems to be the case for honey. Honey has been studied for allergies, and it does not seem to help. In a study of allergy sufferers who routinely had runny noses and irritated eyes from common outdoor allergies, neither local, unfiltered, unpasteurized honey, nor commercially available, filtered, pasteurized honey, improved their allergy symptoms any more than a placebo honey.

Honey is a lovely sweetener, but it is not going to make your allergies go away.

Hot Peppers

Hot peppers can cause ulcers

Constipation isn't the only digestive issue that concerns people enough to make up myths. (See the chapter on cheese if you are worried about dairy and constipation.) Ulcers get their fair share of attention as well. Especially now that gastroesophageal reflux has saturated our consciousness and become a major source of pharmaceutical revenue. Many of us are obsessed with heartburn, and more specifically ulcers.

Ask someone what causes ulcers, and you may hear a number of different things. But most people, when they compile a list, will eventually get around to hot peppers. Like many myths, this one seems to make sense. Hot peppers are, well, hot. They burn your mouth. They can actually cause pain. And so it doesn't seem like much of a leap to assume that they must be causing damage further down as well. It makes sense that, just as they feel like they are burning your mouth, they could be burning the lining of your stomach, causing an ulcer.

It's just not true, though. To understand how this myth, like so many others, is the exact opposite of truth, we have to start with why hot peppers are hot. The heat you feel when you eat them is due to a substance called capsaicin. It has no odor, and it has no taste. Capsaicin is mostly found in the seeds and ribs of peppers, but it is also in the flesh of peppers as well. And when it comes into contact with the nerves in our digestive system, it definitely causes a reaction.

It's important to recognize that this reaction is with the nerves, however. Just because something makes a nerve fire does not mean that it is affecting other cells in any way, certainly not in a bad way. In fact, capsaicin might be doing a lot of good. Studies have shown that capsaicin actually inhibits acid secretion in the stomach. It does not make you have more acid in your stomach (which could cause more ulcers or heartburn): capsaicin makes you have less acid! It also stimulates the secretion of more alkaline substances, which make the stomach even less acidic. It can also stimulate mucus secretion and mucosal blood flow in the stomach, which would act to help prevent or even heal ulcers. Capsaicin does a whole lot more good than harm with respect to ulcers.

Granted, much of this work has been done in rats and not humans, but it's pretty convincing. Moreover, when you have good evidence that there might be protective effects, and no evidence that there are harmful effects, then claiming that something is bad for you is a myth.

As long as we're on the subject, in recent years there has been a flurry of evidence that capsaicin might have other benefits as well. Capsaicin in creams has shown real promise for pain relief. There are promising leads showing that it might slow or stop the replication of prostate cells, which could be helpful for prostate cancer. It's even been helpful in killing human pancreatic cancer cells in mice.

All of this needs further study. And, of course, hot peppers aren't for everyone. That's perfectly acceptable. We just can't stand by and allow the perfectly healthy, and maybe even helpful, hot pepper be unfairly maligned and accused of being harmful.

Hydrogen Peroxide

Hydrogen peroxide is good for a wound

We want to say right off the bat that being concerned about the cleanliness of a wound is a good idea. You want your wounds to be clean. Washing them out is an excellent way to prevent infection. Washing them out with hydrogen peroxide, however, isn't such a good idea. We know you've heard that it is an excellent antiseptic for wounds, but that, unfortunately, is a myth.

We know you are shocked. After all, many of you have used hydrogen peroxide. Hydrogen peroxide has been put on many a skinned knee or cut finger. You've seen it bubble and froth on the cut, which, you've been told, is how you know it's working. It's killing the germs, right there before your eyes. If only it were so.

There have been a number of well-designed studies that have examined how hydrogen peroxide works as an antiseptic. In 1987, in the *Journal of Family Practice*, a randomized controlled trial was conducted comparing topical antibiotics, antiseptics, and wound protectants on their ability to heal wounds. Forty-eight (daring) people volunteered to have six blisters inflicted on them, three on each arm, in such a way that they were infected with a bacteria called *Staphylococcus aureus*. Five different substances were placed on five different blisters, and the sixth was left alone. All the wounds were covered with occlusive dressings. Wounds treated with antibiotic ointments healed significantly faster than any other preparation, and were the only ones that had the infection cleared after two applications. Hydrogen peroxide didn't do that. It did not help to clear the staph infection.

Another study, published in 2009 in the *Journal of Trauma*, exposed cultures of cells to a number of antiseptic solutions to see how they affected cell migration. They found that hydrogen peroxide actually hurt the healing process, by reducing both the migration and proliferation of fibroblasts, which are essential to wound healing. Remember that bubbling? It's the hydrogen peroxide attacking your own cells as much as it is attacking anything infectious. The good cells are not able to come in and do the healing work that they are supposed to.

Adding insult to injury, a paper in the *Journal of Plastic, Reconstructive & Aesthetic Surgery* in 2010 reported on a woman who suffered from a heart attack that seemed to be brought on by an oxygen embolism that was caused by irrigation of a wound on her breast with hydrogen peroxide. Hydrogen peroxide killed her! We're not suggesting this is common or likely to happen, but, as the authors of that report note, it should be factored into decisions that debate the pros and cons of using hydrogen peroxide. Let's recap. Hydrogen peroxide does not appear to help prevent or treat infection in wounds. Hydrogen peroxide does appear to slow healing, and perhaps to cause cell damage. Other antiseptic solutions do appear to promote healing and fight infection. Continuing to believe that hydrogen peroxide is a good thing to use in a wound means continuing to believe in a myth.

Ice

If you cut off your finger, put it on ice right away

We are always amazed at how prepared some people are for the most bizarre kinds of injuries. Take cutting off a finger, for example. Ask a group of people what to do if this happens, and the vast majority will tell you that you should put the finger on ice right away.

First of all, why is everyone so fixated on the finger? You should be much more concerned about the person who lost the finger. Job one, every time, is to make sure the rest of the body (the actual person) is okay. Stabilize the person, make sure he or she isn't bleeding profusely or in shock, and get them help if they need it. Then worry about the finger.

It is worth trying to protect the finger. The technology of surgery has improved such that fingers can still be reattached for up to twelve hours in a regular environment, and for much longer if cooled. Larger limbs with more muscle cannot last quite as long.

You should never give up hope. In 2005, a woman tied up her boyfriend to his bed. Then she cut off his penis and flushed it down the toilet. When rescue people responded, they pulled up the toilet from the floor, and found the penis trapped in an S curve in the pipes. And they still managed to reattach it. You have to love modern medicine.

After you have determined that the person who lost the finger is okay, by all means save the finger. Clean it off. But do not place it directly in ice. If you do so, it's possible that parts of the finger could freeze. If that happens, then the tissues can be damaged in such a way that repair is impossible. For this reason, you should never, ever put a finger in dry ice either. That is way too cold.

Reputable sources recommend that the ideal way to save the finger is to wrap it in sterile gauze and soak it with saline. Then place the wrapped finger in a sealed plastic bag. That bag can be placed in ice. In the likely chance that you don't have these materials, then you can wrap the finger in available cloth, wet it with water, and put that in a sealed plastic bag—which you can cool in ice. It's important that the finger not be in direct contact with the ice, though. You don't want it to freeze.

As always, it's a good idea to be in contact with rescue services in an emergency situation. Not only will they help you get the person and finger to the appropriate facilities as soon as possible, but they will also be able to remind you of the necessary information in order to help both.

Immune System

If you catch a cold, it means you have a weak immune system

In some circles, catching a cold is a sign of weakness. Only those with a weakened immune system are thought to be susceptible to colds. So if you come down with something, it is considered a sign that something is wrong with your immune system.

This is not true! First of all, researchers have done many studies where they try to infect people with colds. They put various viruses that cause colds (rhinoviruses, respiratory syncytial viruses, coronaviruses, and so on) directly into the nostrils of healthy volunteers, and then they see who gets sick and who does not. Under normal conditions, with a normal mix of volunteers, many of the people who are exposed to a cold-causing virus will get sick. When you have cold viruses right in your nose, 75 to 90 percent of those exposed will get sick. That means that lots of normal, strong people still get sick when they are exposed to a nasty virus. People with certain immune deficiencies or disorders of their immune system are, indeed, even more likely to get sick, but most people who get colds do not have problems with their immune system. In one study where 394 healthy subjects had cold viruses put right into their noses, there was no difference in the immune systems of those who got infected and those who stayed healthy when they measured things like while cell counts and total immunoglobulin levels.

Another important thing to remember is that it is normal to get quite a number of colds. Children, in particular, frequently get colds. It is normal for a child to have six to ten colds a year, and that seems like a great deal to parents and everyone involved, but it is normal. Having that many colds does not mean that there is a problem with the child's immune system. Adults do not get quite as many colds either; they get two to four colds a year on average. But it is normal for adults to continue to be exposed to new strains of viruses or to new viruses altogether, and we quite commonly get sick from them. Even if our immune systems are perfectly normal.

That study of 394 volunteers exposed to colds did reveal a different, interesting fact about who was more likely to get sick: having more psychological stress was associated with an increased risk of getting a cold. The more psychological stress a volunteer had, the more likely they were to get infected with the cold virus. Other factors that could have explained the connection between stress and getting sick did not explain it away: in this study, smoking, how much alcohol you drank, your exercise, your diet, how well you slept, and the measures of your immune system did not change whether you got infected compared to your psychological stress. Personality did not matter either. Your level of self-esteem, your personal control, and whether you were introverted or extroverted did not change how likely you were to be infected; it was just your level of psychological stress. It is important to note that smoking by itself renders you significantly more susceptible to colds as well. Based on this study, being under psychological stress does not weaken your immune system in the obvious ways; it does not decrease how many white blood cells you have to fight infections or change the levels of antibodies against infections. But, somehow, those under psychological stress did get infected with colds more often.

While a weak immune system is not to blame, there are a number of interesting factors that are associated with being more susceptible to colds. Psychological stress is one, as we have mentioned. Another issue is not sleeping for very long or not having good quality sleep. People who have a more diverse social network, meaning that they have more friends, family, and work connections, are also less likely to develop colds. How these factors work are not exactly known. The studies are not cause-and-effect studies that tell us how these factors could help or hurt our bodies' susceptibility to colds. Nonetheless, getting enough sleep and trying to decrease stress might be helpful in protecting yourself from colds.

Lice

You can only get lice from another person with lice

The mere mention of lice makes our heads start itching. As pediatricians, we often see children in our clinics with lice, and it never fails to make us start scratching our own heads when we leave the room. You may remember the days in school when someone in the class had lice, and then everyone in the class had to have their heads examined closely for the foul louse. Rachel had very long hair, which was a nightmare for the thorough lice checkers.

Lice are tiny creepy, crawling bugs that live on the head or the hair of the head. They can be tough to see because they are gray or brown and only an eighth of an inch long. The grown-up lice lay eggs that are called nits. These nits or eggs may look like loose white dandruff or flakes in someone's hair, but they are actually stuck very tightly to the strands of hair and do not wash off easily. Lice are baby-making machines. A female louse lives for only thirty days, but she can lay more than 2,600 eggs! Female lice can actually store sperm inside themselves, so mating just once allows them to lay fertilized eggs for their entire lives.

Lice can definitely spread through direct contact with someone else who has head lice. If your head touches the head of a person with lice, their lice can happily—for them—move onto your head and set up camp in your hair. Head lice do not jump or fly, so for a long time people thought that this kind of direct contact was the only way that lice moved from one person to another. Lice require human beings in order to stay alive, and many people have thought that only the adult lice were strong enough to infect another person.

Unfortunately, you can also get lice even if you do not come into direct contact with an infected person's head. You can get lice from sharing a comb, hat, headband, or any other hair accessory with someone who has lice. You can get lice from baseball caps, earphones, pillowcases, and upholstered furniture. Both teenaged lice (called nymphs) and adult lice can live for up to three days when they are not on human beings. The eggs can survive and still hatch into more lice for ten days. (Rachel is scratching her head just contemplating these numbers.) Scientists have tested whether lice can transfer from a scenario where a single strand of hair touches a louse that is on a suspended thread of the sort that you would have on an upholstered chair or a pillowcase. The louse can do it! Another study examined whether lice could be transferred from pillowcases. This study found that, while some lice did move onto the pillowcase at night, only a small number did so. It is possible for the lice to get on the pillowcase and subsequently infect a new person, but it is a much less common way to get infected than being in close contact with someone's head or comb. Even though the risk of being infected from a pillowcase is low, the number of lice that did transfer onto the pillowcases pointed to the need to change pillowcases so you are not reinfected with lice and so that other people are not infected. Lice can be killed from pillowcases by immersing the pillowcase in hot water, by washing in hot water, or by fifteen minutes in a hot clothes dryer.

Lice also have a natural instinct to move quickly away from the light or to move when the hairs in which they are living are disturbed. This makes them very quick at finding new places where they can live, even if that new place is farther away from their original head of hair. Studies of lice movement also find lice crawling on the pillows of people with lice or on the towels of people with lice who have just shampooed, washed, and dried their hair. Combing the hair of someone with lice with a normal comb leaves lice on the comb, on the ground, and on the clothing of the person who does the combing. Hair blow-dryers can also send lice flying into the air, where they can land on other people or on fabrics where they wait around for new people to infect. You can vacuum lice up with a regular vacuum cleaner, but hand vacuums do not pick up all the lice and nits, which can then cause more infestations. Because of how lice spread and flee onto whatever surface they can, most school nurses (who often deal with a lot of lice issues) recommend vacuuming the floors and furniture that have been in contact with someone with lice.

Because lice are so incredibly infectious, it can be really hard to get rid of them, especially once someone in your house has them. Getting lice does not mean that you are dirty or living in bad conditions; it just means that these wily little buggers made a successful attack on your head. To get rid of lice, your best bet is to use a special shampoo designed to kill lice, and then to comb the hair with a special comb designed to help get rid of the sticky nits attached to the hairs. You should consult your doctor about which medicated shampoo to use, especially since some are not safe for young children or pregnant women. In addition to the rounds of shampooing and combing, a lot of cleaning has to go on! Because lice and their eggs can survive on things like pillowcases and hats, you should launder everything that the infected person might have come in contact with. This means washing their bedsheets and towels, and vacuuming all the floors, carpets, and upholstery in the house.

Marriage

Marriage makes you healthy

From as far back as the 1850s, studies of married people versus single people seem to show that you are much better off if you are married. In study after study, married people have been found to be healthier. They seem to live longer, to be less likely to get cancer or to have a heart attack, to get sick less often, and to heal faster than single people. In a meta-analysis that combined the results of marriage studies for more than 250,000 elderly people, those who were widowed, divorced, or single were all at a higher risk of death than those who were married. Changes in marital status, such as becoming widowed or getting a divorce, have been associated with having more health problems in many studies. Marriage seems like a key to good health. In fact, the U.S. government's Healthy Marriage Initiative cites a huge number of benefits from healthy marriages—everything from being physically and emotionally healthier, to having more stable employment and higher wages.

Before you race out to get married or decide that you need to stay married no matter what, you need to understand an important principle behind all of these studies—it matters a great deal whether the marriage is a healthy one or not. A *New York Times* columnist (and one of our favorite health journalists), Tara Parker-Pope, has catalogued the many studies of marriage and health in her book *For Better: The Science of a Good Marriage*. As she summarizes from the many studies, being married alone is not enough to make you healthy. It matters very much whether your marriage is a healthy and happy one. If a person is in a troubled or stressful marriage, he or she is actually less likely to be healthy than a person who was never married at all. A change in your marital status can also lead to more significant health problems; in a study following close to 9,000 men and women, people who became divorced or had a spouse die were more likely to have health problems than people who had never been married.

The quality of the marital relationship matters more than whether you are married. Not only are people in troubled marriages in poorer health than people in strong marriages, but individuals in a troubled marriage have greater health risks than those who are divorced. For example, studies of marital stress and health have found that the immune systems of women in unhappy relationships do not respond as well as the immune systems of women in happy relationships or women who have happily left a relationship. Another study shows that married couples who argue with each other were connected with slower healing of physical wounds on their skin, with the slowest healing for couples who argued with the most hostility. Being in a bad marriage can physically hurt your heart; women with more marital stress are at higher risk of having heart attacks, and married men who have high-conflict fights with their spouses have worse scores on certain heart health ratings. The effects of marital strain also appear to affect a person's health more as people are older. In other words, being in a stressful marriage is more likely to have an even worse effect on your health as you get older. This is another argument against sticking it out in a troubled marriage for any supposed health benefits.

The summary of the current studies of marriage is that marriage can be a great thing for your health—if the marriage is a healthy one! Any unhappy marriage can actually make your health worse, and you should not try to stick it out in a problematic relationship just because you think it will be good for your health. Sadly, the very opposite may be true.

Masturbation

Masturbation will make you go blind

There seem to be as many warnings about masturbation as there are supposed cures for the common cold. (That means there are a lot!) Masturbation is thought to harm you in all sorts of ways. Masturbation will make you go blind. Masturbation will make you grow hair on your palms. Masturbating too much will make you go crazy. Masturbation will make you impotent later in life. Masturbation will make your penis curved. Masturbation will make you unable to have orgasms during regular sex. You shouldn't need to masturbate if you are in a relationship with another person. Masturbation will make you not a virgin. Masturbation will sap your strength. All of these ideas are myths!

One of the most famous proponents of these masturbation myths was none other than the creator of Kellogg's Corn Flakes. Dr. John Harvey Kellogg was a nutritionist and talented surgeon who revolutionized what Americans eat for breakfast. He also happened to be very opposed to sex. Although he was married, he seems to have been abstinent throughout his marriage. Dr. Kellogg was especially against masturbation. He thought masturbation not only caused all of the usual terrible things like blindness and impotence, but also tuberculosis, epilepsy, heart disease, personality changes, and acne. In fact, Dr. Kellogg thought that eating healthy food like Corn Flakes would make people masturbate less. Dr. Kellogg may have been smart about creating breakfast foods, but he was not so smart about masturbation. Eat all the Corn Flakes you want; it is not going to change your masturbating practices.

The evidence that masturbation will not make you blind or make hair grow on your palms is overwhelming. Lots and lots of people masturbate. In fact, even back in the 1940s, 94 percent of males and 40 percent of females reported having masturbated to orgasm. These numbers have only increased, with the percentage of females reporting that they have masturbated at 70 percent or more. In one study in the United States, half of American women reported using a vibrator. It is normal to masturbate. And yet, while lots and lots of people are masturbating, not many people in the world are blind. Even fewer people grow hair on their palms. While mental illness is a real and common problem, it has no connection with masturbation. If masturbation really caused any of these problems, you would see lots and lots of blind, hairy, crazy people all around you. It just does not happen.

Even people who masturbate more than the average do not have physical problems from their masturbation. Researchers have looked closely at people who masturbated an average of four or more times a day over the course of years, and they were not any more likely to have any diseases than the people who masturbated less. Men who ejaculate more often are not going to run out of sperm or become impotent. People who masturbate do not need to worry about their performance in sports or other feats of strength. Having sex or masturbating does not change how well you do on a treadmill and does not seem to change your strength, balance, reaction time, or aerobic power.

Masturbation is not going to deform your penis either. Many men have curved penises or penises that are not perfectly straight. This is completely normal and has nothing to do with whether or not they masturbate. It should not have any negative impact on their experience of sex, although we would recommend talking with a doctor if you have a specific concern about any part of your anatomy.

Masturbation can be a perfectly normal, healthy practice whether you are in a relationship or not. Giving yourself sexual pleasure can be an important way to practice sex, and it is probably the safest form of sex. Knowing what gives you pleasure can also lead to experiencing more pleasure with your partner. Masturbating should not ruin you for sex with another person. It can be a good alternative to sex with someone else, or it can be a healthy way to supplement your sexual relationship with your partner.

Mercury

Your amalgam or metal fillings will make you sick

Mercury has gotten such a bad rap in recent years that it's hard to remember why it was ever considered good in the first place. Though there's no real evidence showing it's a problem, people don't like the mercury in vaccines. There's the mercury in fish, which no one likes. And there's plain old mercury in a number of work sources that causes neurotoxicity, and absolutely no one likes that. So it's no wonder that we finally got around to being upset about the mercury in our dental fillings.

Why is it there in the first place? Well, dentists use it because it works. A dental amalgam filling is 52 percent mercury and 48 percent copper, zinc, and silver. Mercury, an odd metal that is in liquid form at room temperature, binds the other particles together into a tough, long-lasting compound.

So what's the problem? Well, the reason that so many people are concerned about mercury is that there is a fairly large amount of research that shows it's terrible for you. Mercury toxicity has been linked to fatigue, memory loss, and depression. It's also bad for the immune system, and has been shown to interfere with the production of immunoglobulins and antibodies in animal studies. And the fact that mercury got tied into the whole vaccine mess didn't help.

But what makes this a myth is the fact that, while mercury is bad for you, it is much harder to say that the mercury in your fillings is bad for you. For one thing, it is a different kind of mercury. For instance, the mercury in fish is methylmercury, which is an organic mercury. Methylmercury is mostly absorbed in the digestive system and is much more toxic than, for instance, mercury vapor. Mercury vapor is absorbed mostly in the lungs. The mercury in amalgam fillings is elemental mercury, and—you guessed it—it's released as mercury vapor.

Moreover, there are simply no good studies proving that people with mercury amalgam fillings have worse health outcomes, like those above, than those without. And it's not as though those studies would be difficult to do. There are many millions of people with amalgam fillings in their mouths right now. Aaron's got one. Rachel's got many. And any proof of Aaron's superiority cannot be blamed on Rachel having more amalgam fillings.

In fact, such a study has been performed. Scientists looked at two different databases: (1) ninety patients who were part of a clinical trial that removed amalgam fillings in people who thought their health complaints were due to the fillings, and (2) 116 patients from an environmental medicine clinic who thought their symptoms were due to environmental sources, and not the fillings. They found that the amalgam-blaming group more frequently reported mental symptoms while the environment-blaming group had more physical symptoms. Overall, there was no proof of an amalgam-specific syndrome.

Nonamalgam fillings are much more expensive. Many patients simply can't afford them. And fillings are really important to dental health. There are lots of studies that show that having good teeth is a very important part of being healthy overall. People are much better off getting amalgam fillings than nothing, and amalgam fillings are not proven to be bad for your health.

Eating fish while you are pregnant will give your baby birth defects

Most pregnant women want to do whatever it takes to have the healthiest baby possible. Many women quit smoking and avoid drinking alcohol. (And, as pediatricians, we should quickly note that not smoking and not drinking alcohol are proven to be very good ideas for your growing baby!) Pregnant women also try to choose foods that will be safe and healthy for their developing baby. They are instructed to avoid deli meats, sushi, and soft cheeses because of the potential for these foods to harbor dangerous bacteria. They are also told to avoid eating fish because it can contain too much mercury and other toxins.

Whether or not pregnant women should eat fish is a dilemma. Exposure to too much mercury can cause problems for the development of a baby's brain. Too much mercury is not good for any human being, but it is especially problematic when a baby is in the womb and their brains are still developing. Many people have been worried about a connection between being exposed to mercury and developmental delays. While the science on this connection is not conclusive, the concerns make people understandably eager to avoid taking in too much mercury. Fish and shellfish can contain mercury, and so many pregnant women are told to avoid eating them. Even if the risks are relatively small, it makes sense to be extra careful to protect a developing baby.

Eating fish may also impact how big the baby grows. Eating lean fish is also associated with a lower risk of having a baby that is smaller than they should be (this is a good thing). In contrast, eating more servings of canned tuna and shellfish have been associated with a higher risk of having babies that are smaller than they should be. Whether this is related to the amount of mercury in canned tuna or shellfish or whether it is related to something else about these types of fish has not yet been figured out.

Eating fish can be beneficial for both pregnant women and their developing babies. Fish is a good source of protein and contains lots of omega-3 fatty acids, which are considered healthy for our hearts and brains. A review of the research about fish and shellfish that was published in 2006 in the *Journal of the American Medical Association* found that eating more fish was associated with many good things for your body; eating more fish was connected with having less heart disease, fewer deaths from heart disease, and fewer deaths overall. (Perhaps we should recommend a fish a day instead of an apple!) In contrast, the risks from mercury and the other toxins in fish were found to be very low in the studies that were identified. Given the strong benefits from fish and the low risks, this review recommends that even pregnant women should eat fish.

Recent studies have gone even further. They not only find no increase in birth defects among the children of mothers who ate fish, but also that the children of pregnant women who ate fish actually have better scores on tests of their brain development when they are four years old. Even if too much mercury has a potential to cause problems for developing babies, the benefits of fish for the brain may outweigh the risks!

If you want to get the benefits from fish while keeping your risk of mercury poisoning as low as possible, you can eat fish that are extra safe. Some fish contain a lot more mercury than other types of fish. This can also vary from one region to another, so you might want to check what fish are available and recommended where you live. The general recommendations from the United States Department of Health and Human Services state that pregnant women should avoid the fish that have the highest levels of mercury. This means avoiding shark, swordfish, mackerel, and tilefish. The department also recommends that you should not eat more than six ounces of white tuna, albacore tuna, or tuna steak per week. In one week, a pregnant woman should not eat more than two servings or twelve ounces of fish. In general, good fish choices for pregnant women are shrimp, salmon, pollock, catfish, and light tuna, and there may be other fish in your area that are recommended.

Milk

A glass of warm milk will put you to sleep

Warm milk is one of the first recommendations for insomnia. If you cannot sleep, a glass of warm milk is supposed to have you snoozing away in no time. Over a thousand years ago, even the Talmud recommended drinking milk to help you sleep. Many people continue to believe that warm milk will get them snoring quickly. In one study, a third of elderly patients who had tried something to help them sleep in the last year reported that they drank milk to try to get to sleep. Warm milk is one of the most common strategies people use to battle their insomnia.

Unfortunately for the exhausted insomniacs reading this book in the middle of the night, there is no scientific evidence that warm milk will help you sleep. While some patients report that milk helps them sleep, there are no studies showing any benefit in terms of how long it takes to fall asleep or for how long one sleeps.

Some people claim that warm milk is a great cure for insomnia because milk contains tryptophan. You may know that turkey contains tryptophan, and many people blame this substance as the reason why turkey makes you sleepy. Both milk and turkey do contain tryptophan, but you cannot blame the tryptophan from either one for putting you to sleep. (If you read our book, *Don't Swallow Your Gum!*, you may remember that turkey does *not* make you sleepy.) Neither milk nor turkey contains exceptional amounts of tryptophan. Turkey contains about the same amount of tryptophan per gram as ground beef or chicken—0.24 gram of tryptophan per 100 grams of the food. Eggs and cheese contain much more tryptophan per gram than turkey, at 0.3 to 1 gram of tryptophan per gram of food. And milk? A mere 0.08 gram of tryptophan per gram of milk. Not much at all! You need much more tryptophan than that to put you to sleep. An egg and cheese sandwich would be a better bet for the tryptophan, but even with that you would need to eat a lot of sandwiches to get enough tryptophan to have an effect. Moreover, tryptophan is not absorbed well with food. Other people claim that milk somehow changes how tryptophan is absorbed by the body, but there is no science to support that milk helps you sleep by changing how different types of tryptophan are absorbed.

What does work to help you sleep? One of the more effective ways to help you sleep without taking drugs is to use stimulus control therapy. In this technique, you try to retrain yourself to associate the bed with being sleepy. If you are unable to sleep within twenty minutes, you are supposed to leave the bedroom and return only when you are very sleepy. You also avoid doing things like reading or watching television in bed. The only thing you are supposed to do in bed is sleep there. This could actually become one of the ways that milk would work to help someone sleep. If one believes strongly that warm milk makes you sleepy, then this might become a strong enough association in your own mind that milk will help you feel sleepy. Relaxing your muscles slowly, one by one, has also been found to be an effective technique to help you sleep.

Neti Pots

**I have just the thing for that cold . . .
Neti Pots**

Neti pot devotees are a dedicated bunch. After all, it takes a certain level of commitment to fall in love with a "nose bidet" that squirts salt water into your nostrils to wash out your nose and sinuses. Using neti pots began as part of the yogic and ayurvedic traditions. Among those who recommend using neti pots for colds, allergies, and sinus problems are Dr. Oz and Oprah. It is hard to imagine many other people with enough influence to get people to appear willingly on national television with water draining out of their nostrils. Their endorsements made neti pots a popular seller.

The principle of the neti pot is that you irrigate or wash out the nose with sterile salt water (also called saline). This can be done through the use of liquids (like the neti pot bidet) or through non–neti pot methods like drops or a nasal spray. Using salt water to wash out the nose is thought to help sinus conditions or colds by clearing out excess mucus, reducing congestion, and improving your ability to breathe. Salt water washes may help keep your cilia moving to clear mucus and junk out of your respiratory tract. Cilia are little hairlike protrusions on the inside of your respiratory tract that move back and forth to clear things out of your respiratory tract by sending mucus up and out. The other proposed benefits of the neti pot are that it clears out any remaining infectious material from the sinuses and reduces the cough you have from your mucus.

Scientists have tested neti pots for coughs and colds. There have been three good studies done to assess whether cleaning out the nose with salt water improves the symptoms of upper respiratory tract infections, such as nasal discharge, congestion, sneezing, or headache. In these studies, high-concentration or normal-concentration salt water washing is compared to options such as phenylephrine drops (a decongestant), to no treatment, or to usual management for cough and colds such as encouraging the patient to rest, drink fluids, and using whatever medicines they wanted, including anti-fever medicines, antihistamines, and decongestants. The studies of using neti pots for adults and children with colds did not show any significant difference in the symptoms people experienced based on whether they used neti pots. There was no difference overall in the symptom scores that people reported when using the neti pot or other nose-washing methods, and the time it took for cold symptoms to go away was no better. The news for the neti pot was not all bad, though. In one study, the nose washing did improve the respiratory symptoms reported on the first day that it was used, although it did not show any difference after three days of treatment. In another study, people who washed out their noses did not take as much time off work. For children, benefits for the internal nose-washing were not found, and, not surprisingly, children were less willing to use the nose bidet. In summary, neti pots and other ways to wash out the nose do not do much for colds. You might feel more willing to go back to work after using one, but they do not make a big difference over the course of a cold, and may not make any difference at all.

Even though the neti pot is not the solution for your cold, there are problems that the neti pot may actually help with. In a study using daily salt water nose-washing for adults with sinusitis, the patients who used the neti pots reported fewer sinus symptoms and used less antibiotics. One challenge with this study, though, is that the comparison group was not using a fake neti pot or some sort of placebo therapy. It was very easy for everyone to know whether they were using the nasal-washing or not, and that could bias how people think they are feeling or whether they want to use an antibiotic. In interviews of people who used nasal-washing, they reported feeling empowered by being able to do something about their sinus symptoms as well as feeling that the therapy improved their symptoms. How these beliefs alter the results that someone would report in a study will not be known unless we can create a study where people do not know whether they received a neti pot treatment or not.

While the neti pot is unlikely to make any difference for your cold, it is possible that you might sense an improvement in your symptoms if you use a neti pot for sinusitis or long-term sinus symptoms that go on for weeks or months. But if you are not excited about the idea of washing out your nose with salt water, you are probably not missing out on a whole lot.

Nosebleeds

Tilt your head back to stop a nosebleed

Nosebleeds are a pain (sometimes literally). They are inconvenient, messy, and sometimes embarrassing. A commonly given piece of advice is that to stop a nosebleed you should tilt your head back. This advice could not be more wrong.

Sometimes we wish we could just get you to stop what you are doing and seriously think about these myths. Why would tilting your head back help to stop a nosebleed? What effect could it possibly have on the clotting mechanism of the bleed? Does it apply pressure to the wound? Does it restrict blood flow to the lesion? What does it do?

We can think of one thing that tilting your head back might do. It would take the blood that might exit your nostrils and send it streaming down the back of your throat. Now this might seem like a good thing to people around you who are afraid of the sight of blood. It may seem like a good idea to your mother if you're sitting on her clean white couch. And it may seem like a good idea to anyone else who doesn't want to have to deal with your nosebleed.

But it's a terrible idea for *you*. There is a reason that the natural inclination of the blood is to exit your body going forward. That's the safest thing for it to do. Blood heading up your nose and down your throat is a serious choking hazard. It's also possible it will make you vomit. Plus, you might keep bleeding for longer. None of those things is good for you.

Recommendations from reputable organizations are quite clear on what you should do for a nosebleed. First of all, you should keep your head above your heart, so stand, or preferably sit up. Next, you should lean *forward* in order to help the blood drain out of your nostrils and not run down your throat. Some people also recommend that you can apply pressure by squeezing your nose just below the bony bridge for five to fifteen minutes until the bleeding has stopped. Cold icepacks or compresses may also help the nosebleed stop sooner.

Sometimes a nosebleed that won't stop can be an indication that something more serious is at work. You shouldn't hesitate to call for assistance or talk to your doctor if you have recurrent problems with nosebleeds. Of course, you should stop picking your nose first and see if that takes care of the problem.

Oral Sex

You can't get a sexually transmitted disease from oral sex

Safe sex is a very good thing. Unfortunately, many people are uncertain how to have safe sex. While a lot of people know that vaginal sex or anal sex can be dangerous, they think that oral sex is safe.

Oral sex is definitely safer in terms of pregnancy. Giving or receiving oral sex has no risk of getting you pregnant. Getting pregnant requires a sperm to come in contact with an egg inside of a woman. Unless you somehow get some semen in contact with the woman's vagina in the midst of oral sex (Aaron wants to hear how you think that will happen), no one is going to get pregnant.

Getting an infection or a sexually transmitted disease (also called an STD) during oral sex is a possibility, though. You can get an STD from oral sex, whether you are on the giving end or the receiving end, and whether you are male or female. Infections like herpes, gonorrhea, and chlamydia can all spread through oral sex. Both bacteria and viruses can spread from one person to another through oral sex. The virus that causes genital warts and cervical cancer, human papillomavirus (HPV), can even spread through oral sex. The person whose mouth is in contact with the genitals can get infections or sores in their mouth from performing oral sex on someone with one of these infections. And if the person giving oral sex has an infection in their mouth (this is especially common with oral herpes or cold sores), that infection can be passed to the person receiving the oral sex. These infections can be passed even if your partner does not have any symptoms and you do not know that they are infected. (We know this sucks. Pun intended.)

The good news is that most of these infections do not spread as easily through oral sex as they do through vaginal or anal sex. You are much less likely to get herpes, gonorrhea, or chlamydia from oral sex than from these other forms of sex. While it is considered possible to get HIV from oral sex if the person has cuts or sores, experts say it is very unlikely that you would get HIV from oral sex either. Nonetheless, it is possible. Even though it is a low risk, you can get HIV or gonorrhea or herpes from oral sex, especially if there is a cut or sore or something in the person's mouth.

Even if the risks from oral sex are not as high as the risks from other types of sex, the smartest thing is to protect yourself. First, talk with your partner about any infections either of you may have. For men, the penis could be covered with a latex condom. For women, the person giving oral sex could use some sort of protection to create a barrier between the mouth and the vagina. Examples of these kinds of barriers are called a dental dam or a latex sheet, or you could use a condom or even plastic wrap that is cut open to make a protective square. These same things can be used to create a barrier between the mouth and the anus for that kind of oral sex.

We know that the idea of having oral sex with these protective barriers in place does not sound like much fun. However, the idea of getting throat infections, sores in your mouth, or even throat cancers sounds like much less fun. Even worse is the possibility that you could be infected with something like HIV. Play safely!

Oysters

Oysters are an aphrodisiac

Not everyone appreciates the salty, slimy joys of slurping raw oysters, but many people will sample these shelled delicacies just because of their legendary properties. After all, oysters are supposed to get you in the mood and increase your sexual powers.

Rumors of the powers of the oyster go all the way back to the birth of the word "aphrodisiac." Aphrodite, the Greek goddess of love, was born from the sea on an oyster shell and gave birth to Eros. Just as the oyster and the sea gave birth to Aphrodite and Eros, the slippery oyster is supposed to give birth to sexual desire and prowess. In the second century, the Roman satirist Juvenal described how the Romans considered oysters an aphrodisiac food, and even wrote about how women behaved recklessly when they had consumed wine and giant oysters. Legend has it that Casanova, known for his sexual conquests, ate fifty oysters for breakfast every morning to fuel his escapades. Some people think that oysters stay on the list of aphrodisiac foods because they resemble the female genitalia. (Certain foods are believed to fuel sexual appetites because they resemble sexual organs in some way.)

Despite the long-standing reputation of the oyster as a sexual booster, there is no evidence that the oyster has actual powers of sexual rejuvenation. There are no studies documenting increased sexual desire or performance in connection with eating oysters. There is just no science to support the claim that oysters are an aphrodisiac.

Happily for those of us who love oysters, we can still comfort ourselves that they might contain some things that help with sexual performance. Oysters are a good source of zinc, and zinc is needed to make the male sexual hormone testosterone. Having enough zinc in your body is also important to making healthy sperm. Recent studies also suggest that raw oysters contain D-aspartic acid and N-methyl-D-aspartate, two amino acids that increased testosterone levels in a study of male rats. An increase in testosterone levels could result in a boost to your libido. Remember, oysters have never been proven to make any difference in sexual drive, but there is nothing wrong with hoping that they might keep your sperm healthy and your libido strong.

In fact, it is that hope which is likely responsible for the continued belief in the oyster as an aphrodisiac. When we believe that something works, it sometimes does just because of our belief. This is called the placebo effect. Our minds are powerful, and when our mind is convinced that something will have a particular effect on the body, we sometimes can see (or think we see) that effect. Sexual desire is strongly influenced by our state of mind. If you believe that oysters are going to rev up your sex drive, you just might find yourself in the mood after slurping down a few of the bivalve mollusks. It was probably your brain that got you in the mood—not the oysters—but you can enjoy that mood nonetheless.

Penises

You can make your penis bigger without surgery

Many men worry that their penises are not big enough. In one study, only 55 percent of men surveyed reported that they were satisfied with their penis size. (In contrast, most women are pretty happy with their partner's penis size: 85 percent of women report being satisfied.) And men worry more about the length than the width.

Into this vortex of concern and feelings of inadequacy come the advertisements for ways to increase the size of your penis without surgery. Pills, creams, vacuum pumps, and special stretches or squeezing exercises are all touted as the surefire way to increase the size of your member (and make you more pleasing to your partner). We suspect you may be as tired as we are of having to delete these messages from our inboxes, but you also may find yourself wondering, "Do any of these things work?" After all, the idea of increasing your penis size without having to undergo something like surgery does seem awfully appealing.

Many pills, herbs, and creams are marketed as the "proven" way to increase your penis size. Many of them claim that they will increase the blood flow to the penis and thereby increase its size. This is just not true. No medications have been proven to increase penis size. While one mixture of herbs was found to increase the pressure within the penis in rats, and thus might be able to make an erection a bit stronger, none of the herbs was proven to make the penis longer. There is just no science backing these pills, herbs, or creams—regardless of what the manufacturers claim!

Vacuum devices are a popular suggestion for increasing the size of your penis without surgery. These devices are used to treat some forms of erectile dysfunction since they can increase the amount of blood in the tissues of the penis and thus create an erection. Many believe that these devices can also be used to increase the size of the penis. The scientific evidence does not back this one up. In a study of thirty-seven men with penises less than 10 centimeters (when stretched out), vacuum devices were used three times a week, for twenty minutes at a time, for six months. At that time, there was no significant difference in the length of the men's penises. Moreover, only one third of the men were satisfied with the procedure. While these vacuums can play a role after surgery on the penis and in certain types of erectile dysfunction, they just do not work to make the penis any bigger.

Another option touted for making your penis bigger is a penile-extending device. One of these devices has been studied in a somewhat scientific way that involved measurements for twenty-three men who wore the penile extender over the course of three months. This device consists of a plastic ring into which the penis is inserted, and the penis is then attached to two metallic rods by a silicon band. The men were supposed to wear the stretching device for several hours a day, increasing from four to six hours in the beginning to nine hours over the course of the three months, and they were supposed to add a half a centimeter to the length of the rods every two weeks. This study did report that the average length of the flaccid penis (not the erect penis) increased by about 1 centimeter over the course of the three months. The girth of the penis did not change. Based on this one small study, it is possible that stretching your penis for three months might increase the length a little, but it is not clear whether this effect lasts or whether this would make any difference when your penis is erect. It is also important to note that stretching the penis with weights may cause permanent damage to the penis.

In between the unproven pills and creams and more significant surgeries, there is the option to have a doctor inject a type of gel that acts as a "filler" to expand the size of the penis. There is some evidence that having a doctor inject a special kind of gel called hyaluronic acid gel can increase the girth of your penis or the size of the head of the penis. In a small study of fifty men in Korea, using this gel to increase the girth of the penis was found to be satisfactory and safe at eighteen months. The increase in girth was about 4 centimeters (remember, that is measured as circumference around the penis). These are not the best data, as it is a small study in one population, but at least this method seems to work. Not surprisingly, this option has a lot of potential bad side effects. Pain, bruising, changes in the color of the penis, depressions or bumps from uneven spread of the gel, and even embolisms or impotence are possible complications.

We have gone through a bunch of nonsurgical ways to try to increase your penis size, but what about surgery? If none of these pills or lotions or exercises or devices works, should you think about taking the plunge with surgery? In the surgery to make the penis longer, ligaments that hold up the penis are basically cut so that the penis can hang lower and look longer. But even surgery might not be the answer for you. In a critical review of the studies of surgeries to increase the size of the penis, penile enhancement surgery is found to cause a 1–2 centimeter increase in the length of the penis (that's about half an inch) and a 2.5 centimeter increase in the girth of the penis (close to an inch wider in circumference). Surgery can make your penis a bit bigger, though not as much as you might think or hope. There are lots of downsides to surgery, though, and the studies of penile enhancement surgery are full of reports of all kinds of unpleasant complications. Problems like deformity of the penis, paradoxical penile shortening (who wants a penis-lengthening surgery to make it shorter accidentally?), disagreeable scarring (scarring of the penis always seems disagreeable), shifting of the injected material, and sexual dysfunction are all reported as frequent problems with this surgery. In fact, patients are so dissatisfied with these surgeries in both the short term and the long term that the critical review actually concludes that patients should be discouraged from trying these surgeries. Not a good endorsement from urologists and plastic surgeons who specialize in these types of procedures!

It is important to take a moment to think about what is normal and what is not. The average length of an erect penis is between five and seven inches. Most penises, no matter how small or how big they might look when they are soft, end up being about this same length when they are erect. You also might be interested to know that the size of a man's penis falls lower down on a woman's list of requirements than you might think. Women consistently rate a man's personality and grooming higher than penis size in terms of what makes him attractive, and 90 percent of women in one study prioritized the width of the penis over length. Being a fit, attentive, responsive partner is much more likely to be attractive to your partner than having a particular size of penis. Finally, if you really want something else to do, you could work on two optical illusions that might make your member look a bit larger. The most important one for your overall health would be to get rid of your belly. A big belly can hide the upper part of the penis and make it appear smaller. Not only will losing your gut make you much healthier, it might make your penis look bigger too! A less important strategy, but one that you still might want to give a go, is to cut your pubic hair down. Having less bushy hair around the base of your penis might create the illusion that your penis is a bit bigger. Once again, your partner may not care at all, but you can try this one out if you want something to work on.

Poison

If you swallow something poisonous, you need to vomit as soon as possible

Finding out your child has swallowed something potentially poisonous can be a harrowing experience. Unfortunately, many people's first instinct is to try and get them to vomit it up. It makes sense, doesn't it? If the poison is bad, get it out of the stomach as quickly as possible.

There are so many reasons that this is a bad idea. First of all, when you vomit up a substance, you seriously increase the chance that it can go into the lungs. This is very, very bad. And, with some substances, like products made from petroleum, the vapor can cause a bad pneumonia. Moreover, sometimes children and adults can have an altered consciousness after swallowing something bad, which can greatly increase the risk of having things go into their lungs that should not.

A lot of things that children unintentionally swallow are very likely to burn their throats. Anything alkaline, including many dish-washing and cleaning products, is likely to chemically burn tissues with which it comes into contact. Vomiting these products increases the exposure to the throat an additional time (while also putting the lungs at risk). Vomiting is a terrible idea with these.

And there are other reasons not to induce vomiting. Vomiting increases the pressure in the stomach, which can increase absorption of stomach contents. You definitely do not want the person to absorb more of what they swallowed. Vomiting, once begun, can be hard to control and stop. Some of the methods to induce vomiting can also be dangerous themselves. People have been known to force the swallowing of salt water, which is not a good idea. Salt water can actually irritate the lining of your stomach and intestines, possibly even making you absorb more of the poison, and too much salt water without other fluids can lead to dehydration. Moreover, using salt water to make someone vomit is a bad idea for many of the same reasons that using ipecac to force vomiting is bad—which we'll get to momentarily. The chemical that was swallowed might cause worse burns as it comes back up, and the vomiting could cause you to aspirate or to breathe in the chemicals or poisons that were swallowed. Shoving your fingers into another's throat can also cause harm.

And all of this ignores the fact that vomiting isn't a particularly good way to completely evacuate or clear out the stomach.

This all brings us to ipecac. Once again, the medical field is partly to blame for perpetuating a medical myth. For decades, we advised parents and families to have a bottle of ipecac on hand, in case we ever wanted a person to induce vomiting in just this situation. The problem is that ipecac doesn't really do any good (for many of the reasons mentioned above), and it can potentially do a lot of harm (again, see above). Ipecac makes people vomit, but there are far too many reasons why vomiting that poison up might be a bad idea.

In a landmark study published in *Pediatrics* in 2003, Dr. Gary Bond showed that in a review of sixty-four U.S. poison centers and over 750,000 calls to poison centers, the use of ipecac did nothing to prevent resource utilization including hospitalizations. It also did nothing to improve patient outcomes at all. Even if you used ipecac, you still had to come to the hospital. And it did not prevent any of the harms that come when you swallow something you should not. The American Academy of Pediatrics, and many other organizations, subsequently changed their recommendations and told people to throw out the ipecac. We would

POISON

advise you to do the same! If you think your child, or anyone else, has swallowed something poisonous or harmful, you should always, and we mean *always*, call a poison control center. The phone number for the national center is 1-800-222-1222.

Protein

Eating extra protein after you work out will help you build muscles

This one is a half-truth. Eating protein does help you build muscles; a process called protein synthesis is key to that. Protein supplements do seem to help people to build bigger, stronger muscles.

In studies in which people are randomized to consume protein supplements or carbohydrate supplements before and after exercise, the people who take the protein supplements do build more muscle mass and have greater muscle strength. Combining protein supplements with resistance training does boost muscle protein synthesis and improve muscle performance in small studies.

However, you don't need to take in huge amounts of protein in order to do this. Experts say that you do not need more than 0.9 to 1.25 grams of protein per pound of body weight. If you take in any more than that, your body will just convert the protein into other things that are stored up for energy or else you will excrete the extra out.

It is also important to remember that eating protein alone is not going to build up your muscles. You need to exercise your muscles AND eat the protein if you are going to see any effects from your bodybuilding. And if you were going to do only one of those things, it would have to be the exercising. Taking in extra protein-based calories is just going to lead to an excess of calories otherwise. The body stores extra calories as fat, not as protein.

The effectiveness of protein supplements needs to be balanced against the risks. Bodybuilders who take in huge amounts of protein can actually create other problems for their body. Too much protein can make the body dehydrated. The kidneys have to work hard to get rid of all the extra, which places an added stress on them. There is evidence that taking a low dose of a supplement such as creatine does not hurt the kidneys, but the long-term effects of taking higher doses of these supplements are not known. Higher-protein diets can also cause digestive problems, such as more gas, indigestion, and heartburn. And regularly eating a high-protein diet has been connected with a higher risk of developing heart disease in some studies.

Saunas

Saunas or sweat lodges will cleanse your body of toxins

Sweat lodges have traditionally been used for religious purposes and purification ceremonies. People continue to go to sweat lodges for a spiritual experience or in an effort to detoxify their body. Saunas are often used for similar purposes; many people find them relaxing, but also hope that the heat and sweating will cleanse their bodies.

Sweating is not the way to release toxins from the body. The main role of sweating is to cool your body. The moisture produced by your sweat glands evaporates, and this evaporation process cools the body. The primary role of sweating is for cooling you off. Water, electrolytes, and some other chemicals are released through your sweat, but detoxifying is not the main role of sweating. Many people don't realize that their sweat glands are not directly connected to other systems in their body, like their digestive track or their lymph nodes.

Sweat is mostly water, but it does contain some other chemicals dissolved in it—minerals (small amounts of sodium, lactate, urea, potassium, calcium, magnesium), trace elements (very small amounts of zinc, copper, nickel, iron, chromium), and some chemicals that smell (2-methylphenol and 4-methylphenol). Sodium (salt) is the most common mineral in sweat and the concentration of sodium in sweat varies based on how hot a person is and how much they are exercising.

Even though sweat has some chemicals in it, you should not

rely on sweating to detoxify your body. Although small amounts of minerals and trace elements are eliminated from the body through sweating, this is not the main purpose of sweating. The purpose of sweating is to cool the body—not to cleanse the body. You mostly just lose water through sweat.

Saunas are not necessarily bad for the body. There is some evidence that saunas improve blood pressure and enhance blood flow and cardiac function. However, the medical literature does not provide very clear scientific evidence of health benefits to sweat lodges, steam rooms, or saunas.

A sweat lodge can be more of a danger than a benefit to your body if proper precautions are not taken. One of the biggest risks is getting overheated. Being overheated can lead to heat exhaustion or more severe problems such as heat stroke or hyperthermia. This is probably what happened recently when several people died after their experience in a sweat lodge in Arizona. Your body always works to try to balance how much heat it makes and how much it loses, but if you are in conditions that are too hot for too long, your body may not be able to cool you off well enough. In addition to feeling thirsty and hot, you may begin to feel dizzy, weak, clumsy, and sick to your stomach. These are signs that you need to move to a cool place, drink fluids, and seek medical care. People with heart conditions should always talk to their doctors before trying a sweat lodge or sauna.

To avoid other risks in sweat lodges, you should not take part in a ceremony where hot river rocks or other rocks with air pockets are used. These rocks can occasionally explode in the heat, injuring people around them. You should also make sure not to wear metal jewelry that could heat up and burn you in very hot conditions.

The body is great at detoxifying itself. Your liver specializes in breaking down substances within the body, including many of the chemicals that your body cannot use or that would be considered toxins. Your kidneys also do a lot of work to get rid of toxic substances like urea—much more work than your sweat glands do. Your entire digestive system, including your colon, is designed to get rid of what your body cannot use and to keep what it needs. Your body does not rely on sweating to keep itself healthy, and neither should you.

Seizures

If someone is having a seizure, you should put something in their mouth

Seizures can be pretty scary for people who aren't used to seeing them. In a typical grand mal seizure, a person or child will lose all voluntary motor control and shake, sometimes violently. Unfortunately, when these seizures are presented in movies or TV shows, invariably someone offers the following advice: "Put something in his mouth so he can't swallow his tongue."

Never, ever do that.

The first thing to do is stay calm. The vast majority of seizures are not life-threatening, and most won't even need medical intervention. So stay relaxed, and reassure those around you. The next thing to do is make sure there isn't anything on the ground that could hurt the person having a seizure if he were to hit it. If there are sharp objects, you should move them away. Don't, however, try to relocate the person. Don't lift someone having a seizure or try and restrain them. They aren't going to hurt themselves. Of course, if they are near a cliff or road, you should prevent them from going over. Common sense should still apply.

It is totally reasonable to loosen a tie or anything around a seizing person's neck. It is also a good idea to turn them gently onto their side so any liquid in the mouth drains out. You can even cushion their head gently as long as you don't restrain them. It's also a good idea to time the seizure; you should get more concerned if it lasts five minutes or more.

What you should never, ever do is pry open a person's mouth

or put anything in it while they are having a seizure. Contrary to what you may have heard, a person cannot swallow their tongue while they are having a seizure. Forcing a person's mouth open could injure their teeth, tongue, or jaw. It could also result in a serious injury to your fingers. Placing anything in their mouth also places them at serious risk for choking.

You should always err on the side of caution when considering calling for help. If you're concerned, call. That's what emergency services are for. But most of the time they aren't necessary. Exceptions include pregnant women, people with diabetes, and seizures that occur in water or last more than five minutes. You should also call if a seizing person stops breathing, starts seizing again before waking up, or if the person comes out of the seizure and says this was his or her first seizure.

Sex

Having sex during pregnancy will hurt the baby

In the movie *Knocked Up*, the main characters are on the brink of reenacting the scenario that got one of them "knocked up" in the first place when the guy becomes paranoid that he cannot have sex with his pregnant romantic interest without doing damage to the baby. Seth Rogen's character is not alone; many people worry about whether sex will hurt their baby, cause a miscarriage, or cause problems in some way for the pregnancy.

There are plenty of real things to worry about during a pregnancy. Whether or not you can have sex is not one of them! Sex during pregnancy is completely safe if the pregnancy is a normal one. The experience of millions of human beings over time should reinforce how true this is. Most women have sex while they are pregnant, and most babies turn out just fine. Nonetheless, scientists have studied this question.

There is no scientific evidence that sex during any stage of pregnancy will hurt the baby or the mother under normal conditions. There is no evidence that sex causes miscarriages. In studies comparing babies born to mothers who had sex throughout pregnancy with babies born to mothers who stopped having sex at some point in the pregnancy, there were no differences between the babies. There were also no differences in the babies born to mothers who had orgasms during their pregnancies and those who did not have orgasms. Sex is usually perfectly safe for the baby and the mother.

While many people believe that sex might cause a miscarriage, especially early in the pregnancy, there is no evidence to support this. Most miscarriages, particular the early ones, result from an abnormality in how the baby is developing or a chromosomal problem. The miscarriage is not related to anything that you have done or not done. Sex will not make a difference. In fact, a recent study suggests that it is better to try to conceive again in the months soon after a miscarriage than to wait six months or more. Sex did not cause the miscarriage, and you can try again quite soon.

Other people worry that sex might not be good for the baby because of just how close the baby and the penis might be to each other. The baby is actually well protected from the penis during sex. Inside the uterus, the baby is surrounded by amniotic fluid, which offers a good barrier. The entrance to the uterus, the cervix, is a relatively thick cap over the uterus with just a small hole in the middle (until the very end of pregnancy when the cervix starts to dilate or open up a bit). The baby is further protected by a mucus plug that seals off the cervix throughout most of the pregnancy as well. The penis is not going to touch the baby.

There are a few circumstances in which sex is not recommended for a pregnant woman. If the woman is having bleeding, significant pain, or leaking amniotic fluid, the doctors will often recommend not having sex. Women with a history of having babies prematurely or with signs of premature labor might also be warned against having sex. Any of these recommendations would be individualized decisions between a woman and her doctor. Moreover, there is not much scientific evidence to support that sex would make any difference in these scenarios, so it is likely a matter of being extra cautious.

There are only two precautions that other pregnant women should be concerned about when it comes to sex. First of all, if they are receiving oral sex, their partner should not blow air into their vagina. In very rare circumstances, this can cause a bubble of air to go into a blood vessel and cause problems for the mother or baby. This is easy to avoid. The other thing that really could be bad for a pregnant woman or baby is if the mother has sex with someone who is infected with a sexually transmitted disease or HIV. You may not be able to tell if your partner has diseases like syphilis and gonorrhea, or HIV, and these can create terrible problems for the baby. These infections and other sexually transmitted diseases can cause birth defects, infect the baby, and sometimes even kill the baby. Safe sex is important during pregnancy to protect the mother and the baby, so use a condom if there is any question as to whether your partner has any infections.

Pregnant women do not always want to have sex. Depending on their fatigue and nausea during the early stages of pregnancy and their general discomfort during the latter stages, woman's interest in sex might fall off. On the other hand, it is important for pregnant women and their partners to know that, if they want to do it, sex is safe and healthy.

You should not have sex or masturbate before a big game

Before a big game or competition, athletes are often warned that they should not have sex. Surveys of coaches and athletes reveal that many believe that pregame sex does or might hurt athletic performance. Legend even has it that amazing performers like Muhammad Ali would not have sex for six entire weeks before a fight. The worry is that sex or masturbation will take too much of your strength or leave you too spent to perform at the peak of your abilities. Many people believe that sexual frustration may also increase your level of aggression or strength. In contrast, having a sexual release is thought to decrease how much testosterone you have.

If you look at the physiology or the science of how the body works, there is no reason to abstain from sex before a big game. In fact, you might actually perform better if you have sex the night before! In one study, men who had sex the night before a sporting event actually had higher testosterone levels the next day. This directly contradicts the fears that having sex would leave you without energy or strength the next day. Ejaculation does not decrease your testosterone levels, and instead seems to enhance it. It is possible that higher testosterone levels would lead to better performances in terms of aggression or strength. Studies have also found that leg muscle strength and flexibility do not get any worse after you have had sex.

Most of the studies of the impact of sex on athletic performance have been done with men, but there is also evidence that sex might improve women's performance. In particular, women who had sex the day before are found to better block the release of a neuropeptide that transmits pain. Experiencing less pain could be a bonus for competitors.

Just how much energy sex might use up before your big game is another matter of mythology. As much as you might like to think that your antics in bed are strenuous exercise, this is not the case for the average person. Most people only use about twenty-five to fifty extra calories when they have sex. They only burn about six calories a minute during sex, and the average sexual encounter does not last as long as you might imagine. Sex takes about as much work as walking up two flights of stairs. Most athletes would never worry about two flights of stairs zapping their strength.

Of course, the effect of sex on the body is not purely a matter of physiology. The brain plays an important role too. There might be psychological or emotional reasons why it would be good to abstain before an important athletic performance. If sex distracts you or takes away the mental focus that is key to your putting in your best game, experts say that sex might then have a negative effect on your performance for psychological reasons.

On the other hand, if sex helps you to have a good night's sleep, it may be just the thing that you need before that competition. The key for the psychological state of any athlete is reaching the right balance between being well rested and being alert, with just enough anxiety to keep you sharp and focused. For some, sex might be an important factor in this equation.

In terms of your strength and hormones, having sex or masturbating before a big game is unlikely to do any harm. Of course, staying awake all night or becoming embroiled in an interaction that leaves you distracted or tense might not be a good idea. The safest strategy is probably to follow your usual routine when deciding what activities ought to make up your pregame evening. And if you need a testosterone boost, this gives you a good excuse for sex!

Sex is bad for your heart

Once a person has had a heart attack, they often worry about whether they will be able to have sex again. Everyone has heard horror stories of people dying of a heart attack in the middle of sex, and those with a history of heart disease may be particularly afraid that sex is going to be too much for their heart. People seem to believe that various sexual antics are particularly strenuous for their heart.

Sex is not bad for your heart! In fact, having sex more often is connected to having a healthier heart. In a study that followed 1,165 men for an average of sixteen years, the men who reported having sex twice a week or more had a lower risk of developing cardiovascular disease (things like heart attacks, strokes, or peripheral artery disease). In contrast, the men who engaged in sexual activity once a month or less had an increased risk of developing cardiovascular disease during the study. The men who had sex less were 45 percent more likely to develop these heart-related problems, and this was unrelated to age or erectile dysfunction. Whether having sex more often was a marker for being in good shape overall or whether it was tied to having a strong intimate relationship, having sex was strongly tied to having a healthy heart.

The chance of having a heart attack while you are having sex is also very low. A large study called the Framingham Heart Study has given us good information on these kinds of risks by following lots and lots of men since 1948 and looking at their risk factors and heart problems. This study tells us that, if you are a man who does not have diabetes and does not smoke, the chance that you will have a heart attack during sex is one in a million! Even if you have heart disease, if you are able to pass a basic stress test, the chance you will have a heart attack during sex only goes up to ten in a million. From another study that looked at the determinants of heart attacks, we have learned that a fifty-year-old man who does not have heart disease and who has an annual risk of 1 percent for having a heart attack will only increase his risk of a heart attack to 1.01 percent if he has sex once a week. In case the numbers are confusing for you, the summary is this: the chance that you will have a heart attack during sex is quite low.

What if your heart has already had problems? One of the big concerns people have about having sex after a heart attack is that it will be too strenuous on their heart. While people who have had a heart attack do need to exercise some caution in terms of resuming normal activities, they do not need to be so afraid of having sex. As we've already pointed out, the truth is that most people just do not exert themselves that much during sex! The physical exertion most people put in when having sex, as we have seen, is similar to walking up two flights of stairs; sex does require some exertion, but it is not like running a marathon. Walking at about four miles per hour on a treadmill—the kind of stress test that heart attack victims will usually have to complete before they leave the hospital—is about the same level of exertion that you would have during sex that produces an orgasm. If you can do the treadmill walking, you are probably ready for sex. While a person who has had a heart attack usually needs to be careful about building up to their previous level of exercise, you will probably be ready for sex much sooner than for other activities. How soon you can resume sex also depends on what you mean by sex. Some sexual activities are more strenuous than others. The best way to know what you should or should not do and how soon you can do it is to talk with your doctor about your individual heart condition and what you would like to do sexually. Patients with particular symptoms or on certain drugs may need to be more careful than others, but your doctor can help you determine what your risk level is.

Moreover, fear itself may be your biggest problem with having sex after a heart attack. If you are too afraid to have sex because you are afraid it will hurt you or your partner's heart, that fear could become the barrier to having healthy, enjoyable sex after a heart attack. This is another reason to talk with your doctor (and your partner) about the real risks involved, but also about the ways in which you can engage in and foster the loving, caring aspects of your sexual relationship.

Sit-ups

Sit-ups or crunches will flatten your stomach

Most of us have had that moment where we look down at our too soft belly and decide that something needs to change. When confronting our undesirable gut, many of us resolve to do more crunches. Sit-ups are considered the key to a flat, hard abdomen. Sadly, the truth is that you might do more sit-ups than you care to count and still have a flabby gut. Why is this?

When you do crunches or sit-ups regularly, you do strengthen and define your abdominal muscles. However, if you are not burning up more calories than you take in, you will not lose fat. And that means that those toned, defined abdominal muscles might still be well hidden underneath a layer of belly fat. Crunches may work the muscles of your abdomen, but they are probably not enough to make you lose the weight you need to in order to let you show them off.

Unfortunately, working the muscles in a particular spot does not mean that you will lose fat from that area. As you've probably heard over and over, spot reduction does not work. Reducing the amount of fat in your body usually requires cardiovascular exercise that increases your heart rate and gets your entire body moving, so that you burn enough calories to tip the balance toward weight loss. For example, a study of obese women found that high-intensity exercise training was the most effective way to eliminate the total fat around the abdomen, as well as the abdominal fat under the skin and the fat around the organs of the abdomen.

It is also difficult to predict or target where on the body a person will lose weight. When scientists study weight loss through restricting calories (dieting), dieting plus engaging in moderate exercise, and dieting plus engaging in vigorous exercise, there is no preferential loss of weight from the abdomen. Among people who lose the same amount of weight, different types or intensities of exercise did not make them any more likely to lose weight from their bellies. While losing weight from anywhere on the body is a good thing if you are overweight, we don't get to pick and choose which areas get smaller.

Another important note related to sit-ups is that they are often not even the best exercise for strengthening your abs. Sit-ups actually engage the flexor muscles in the trunk, specifically the iliopsoas muscles, more than they do the abdominal muscles that would be part of that six-pack you're striving for. The iliopsoas muscles are best thought of as the inner hip muscles, and they actually connect to your lower back. These muscles are important for walking, running, and standing, so it is worthwhile to keep them in good shape, but you may want to consider other muscles when working on toning your abs.

Sneezing

Your heart stops beating when you sneeze

People have believed a lot of scary things about sneezing over the ages. In some traditions, the soul was thought to leave the body when you sneeze, allowing evil spirits to sneak in unless you are protected with a "God bless you." Another belief was that the forceful sneeze actually expelled evil spirits out from the body. Tradition also holds that people began blessing each other after they sneezed because those who were stricken with the plague did a lot of sneezing. Since the plague killed so many people, religious authorities suggested that blessings or prayers should be offered for those who were sneezing. Perhaps the scariest belief that has persisted over time is the idea that your heart stops beating when you sneeze.

Your body operates with an impressive amount of force when you sneeze. Sneezing engages muscles in your face, neck, chest, and abdomen to spew out air and mucus at an average of 100 miles per hour. Your body sneezes in reaction to things that irritate the lining of your nose and upper respiratory tract. Whether it is dust or pollen in the air irritating your nose, or a cold virus multiplying on the inner surface of your nose, these irritants trigger a particular reflex in your body that makes you sneeze. This is one of the ways that your body protects you—whether from invaders or from all the powderlike little things that might otherwise end up in your lungs. In some people, the sneezing reflex can also be triggered by light; people with photic sneezing may sneeze when they walk out into the sunshine or see a very bright light. Scientists do not fully understand how this works, but they think that the light somehow triggers the nerves involved in sneezing by working on your retina in a certain way or by how you squint.

As powerful as sneezes are, and as strange as the mechanisms that trigger sneezes may be, your heart does not stop when you sneeze. The contracting or beating of your heart is controlled by an electrical system that runs through the muscles of the heart wall. The heart's electrical activity is not stopped by sneezing. Your heart keeps beating.

However, sneezing can change how your heart beats. The process of sneezing can actually slow down how fast your heart is beating for a moment, and this change in the heart's rhythm is likely why people believe that sneezing stops their heart. When you sneeze, you take a big breath or inhalation in. This increases the pressure inside your chest. Then, the powerful contracting of your muscles when you sneeze causes the pressure to increase again. These changes in pressure, which combine with changes in blood flow to and from the heart, temporarily slow how fast your heart beats. As the rate changes, you may have the feeling that your heart has skipped a beat or even that your heart has stopped. Your heart never stops; it just slows down a bit.

Starting to feel sniffly? The most important thing to remember about sneezing may be that it sends your mucus up to five or six feet around you, all propelling out at 100 miles an hour. Any germs that are making you sick can really get spread around. So, cover your nose and mouth as best you can, and keep washing your hands!

Snow

Sitting in the snow will give you a urinary tract infection

One of our colleagues is from Sweden, and she swears to us that this is a popular myth over there, which proves two things: first, that no country is immune from believing medical myths, and second, that some health myths are regional. We have found no evidence that this myth is true (or even that it has been studied), and, guess what: it's just not true. You can't catch a urinary tract infection from sitting in the snow.

As long as we have your attention, though, we might as well talk to you about the other myths and truths about urinary tract infections. First off, they are very common. They account for more than eight million visits to the doctor each year, and about 20 percent of women will have at least one over the course of their lives. Urinary tract infections in children are not rare. By the time they are five, almost one in ten girls will have had a urinary tract infection, and 1 to 2 percent of boys will have had one as well.

So what does make you more likely to have a urinary tract infection? The biggest risk factor, by far, is being female. Why? Well, that is simply because it's much harder for bacteria to get into a male's bladder than a woman's. We'll give you a minute to picture the different anatomy and imagine why that's so. See? The penis has so many uses. There is a much longer distance from the tip of a penis to a male's bladder than from the vagina to a female's bladder. Urinary tract infections are pretty uncommon in males, but when they occur they are often serious and an indication that something else is wrong.

Sexual activity increases the risk of a urinary tract infection, as do certain types of birth control, such as diaphragms and spermicidal agents. This is likely due to the fact that you're putting foreign objects close to the urethra, and, well, bacteria on them might infect you. Sorry, but it's true.

Women who have gone through menopause are at increased risk for urinary tract infections because low estrogen levels change the urinary tract in ways that leave it more likely to be infected. People with diabetes or other disorders that can reduce the effectiveness of the immune system can also be at increased risk. Children who have physical abnormalities of the urinary tract are much more likely to develop urinary tract infections.

Now on to things that are not risk factors. Studies have shown that pregnant women are no more likely to get urinary tract infections than women who are not pregnant. However, urinary tract infections in pregnant women, when they do occur, can be more serious as bacteria more often move up to the kidneys from the bladder. This may be due to hormonal changes that occur in pregnancy that make it easier for the bacteria to move.

Another thing that gets a bad rap is bubble baths for children. Pediatricians like us often tell parents not to let children sit in bubble baths because it increases the risk of urinary tract infections in children. However, a good review of the literature found that, while bubble baths might cause some external irritation in the vagina, there is no link proving that they increase urinary tract infections. And kids love bubble baths. So it's just as likely that depriving them of the bubble baths will decrease the likelihood that they might bathe. We want children to bathe!

To recap: anatomical abnormalities, menopause, sex, and being a woman make you more likely to get a urinary tract infection. Pregnancy doesn't make them more common, but does make them more serious. And bubble baths are unfairly maligned. Oh, and by the way, snow has nothing to do with them at all. Sorry, Sweden.

Soap

Using soap is the best way
to clean your hands

One of the most important messages we've tried to get across in this book is that washing your hands is key to avoiding a whole slew of illnesses, especially the common cold. Avoiding cold weather, dressing warmly, and making sure you dry your hair completely before heading outside will not keep you healthy. Neither vitamin C, nor echinacea, nor zinc, nor Airborne, nor Emergen-C will prevent you from catching a cold. Amidst all these things that don't work, hand-washing is a clear winner.

Washing your hands makes you much less likely to be infected with the germs that cause all sorts of nasty problems like diarrhea or colds. In the literature about infections, experts recommend hand-washing time and time again. The general principle is that you should wet your hands with running water, put some soap on your hands, lather up, and then rub your hands together vigorously for at least twenty seconds. (That is a much longer time than you think. We bet it is much longer than you usually wash your hands.) Then you should rinse off your hands and dry them. Hand-washing is recommended after you prepare food, use the toilet, change diapers, touch animals, blow your nose, cough, handle garbage, or touch a sick person.

Many people assume that soap and water are vital when it comes to washing your hands. This is a half-truth. Using soap and water is the classic way to wash your hands, and it does remove much of the bacteria from your hands. However, just having soap and water is not necessarily good enough. Whether the hand-washing is going to protect you depends on the length of time you wash, how much soap you use, what type of soap you use, and how the soap is stored. Soap alone is not enough! The longer you wash, especially when you wash for more than fifteen seconds, the more bacteria you remove from your hands. Using more soap rather than less soap also improves the cleaning abilities, as does using an antimicrobial soap.

However, you cannot put your complete trust in soap. Soap can actually become contaminated with bacteria. Soap contamination has led to outbreaks of infections in places like neonatal intensive care units in hospitals, and bacteria can be cultured from soap in hospitals all around the world. Bar soaps and soaps that are stored improperly, especially in standing water, are more likely to be contaminated. If your only choice for washing your hands is a very dirty bar of soap sitting in grimy water on the edge of a sink, you may be better off skipping the soap altogether and maximizing the other elements of good hand-washing. In such a case, you should use lots of friction between your hands and wash for a long time. Using paper towels instead of the hot air dryer is also a very good idea.

Soap also becomes less important when you consider its competitor—the alcohol-based hand rub. These hand sanitizers have become popular around hospitals, offices, and schools for a very good reason. They work great! In most studies, alcohol-based hand rubs do better than hand-washing with soap and water at removing bacteria from the skin. There are a few types of bugs that cause infection through spores that seem to come off better with very vigorous hand-washing with soap and water, but the hand sanitizers win overall. If your only option is a hand sanitizer and not soap and water, you should be happy the hand sanitizer is actually the better choice. Moreover, not only does the hand sanitizer remove more bacteria from your hands, it is also cost-effective when you compare it to washing with soap and water.

We are still big fans of soap, but soap can't make it on its own. You need to make sure you wash your hands long enough, with enough friction, and with a noncontaminated soap. Plus, using an alcohol-based hand gel or sanitizer may be a better choice.

Solid Foods

**If you wait longer to start solid foods,
your baby won't get as many allergies**

The origins of some myths are difficult to figure out. This is not one of those myths. And, to some extent, we physicians are to blame.

For the first few months of life, the only thing babies are supposed to eat is breast milk or formula. That's it. No water, no juice, no foods. But as babies get older, they have to start eating solid foods. Usually we recommend that they start with cereals around four months of age, progress to vegetables or fruits around six months, and then finally on to more complex foods.

The process by which babies are introduced to new foods has been made more and more complicated over time. You can imagine that mothers long ago did not really think too hard about what foods were introduced or when. But today, we usually recommend starting one new food at a time, and giving that food alone for at least a few days. That way, if the baby is allergic to that food, we can find out in the least confusing manner. If the baby starts several foods at the same time and has a bad reaction, we would not know which food was causing the problem.

This focus on allergies is not limited to when you start foods. For some time, there was a lot of confusion and debate on when to start introducing solid foods. Many believed that delaying the introduction of solid foods would make it much less likely that babies would have allergic difficulties.

Allergies are a pretty big deal. According to the CDC, about

4 percent of children have a food or digestive allergy. Some of these reactions are quite severe. Moreover, children who have food allergies are also much more likely to have other disorders or allergies. So preventing allergies or limiting their development is important.

Unfortunately, the recommendations to delay the introduction of solid foods were not based on good science. In fact, a 2006 systematic review looking at all the studies on this issue concluded that there really was no evidence to support a connection between early feedings of solid foods and asthma, allergic rhinitis, animal dander allergy, or persistent food allergies. (Aaron was actually a co-author of that study.)

Since then, several more well-designed studies have confirmed that there is no link between starting foods early and developing allergies. Many medical organizations have adjusted their recommendations to no longer promote delaying introduction of solid foods to prevent allergies. And, in 2010, a study published in *Pediatrics* found evidence that the late introduction of "potatoes (>4 months), oats (>5 months), rye (>7 months), wheat (>6 months), meat (>5.5 months), fish (>8.2 months), and eggs (>10.5 months)" was actually linked to an increased risk of developing allergies.

As always, you should talk with your pediatrician about the best time to introduce solid foods for your baby. There is no one correct answer for every baby, and it is a personal decision. You and your doctor should know, however, that delaying the introduction of solid foods in order to prevent food allergies is a myth.

Sponges

Wiping everything with a sponge will keep the bathroom or kitchen clean

If reading about all the germs in your house does not inspire you to start cleaning, we don't know what will. But before you go and do so, you should seriously consider how you will do so. Many of you use a sponge to clean in the bathroom or kitchen. Sponges are certainly common cleaning tools and seem like a good weapon to attack all of those bugs, spills, and stains. Is this a good idea, though?

Likely no. You see, contrary to what you might think, sponges become contaminated with germs when they wash things. The more things you wash, and the longer you use the sponge, the dirtier it gets. Soon, it starts transferring germs to other surfaces.

There's research to back this up. In a study published in 2002 in the *International Journal of Food Microbiology*, scientists specifically examined how germs found in food moved around the kitchen during cleaning. One part of the study looked at how germs were transferred from a sponge to surfaces in the kitchen. They found that, on average, wiping a 20x30 centimeter surface clean transferred less than a gram of liquid. However, depending on the concentration of bugs in previously washed items, both salmonella and E. coli could be transferred from the sponge to other surfaces in the kitchen.

Another study examined what items in the home had germs on them. Items with what was deemed a "high" count included drain traps (91 percent), sinks (67 percent), and, yes, sponges (78 percent). The germs detected included such horrors as E. coli, *Staphylococcus aureus,* and *Pseudomonas aeruginosa.* Sponges in the bathroom were also noted to have high counts of bacteria. For comparison purposes, the percentage of toilet seats or bowl rims with high counts were only 1 to 2 percent. It's crazy. The toilet is probably cleaner than your sponge!

So what can you do? Well, there have actually been studies of methods to clean sponges. They include rinsing, bleach, and putting them in the dishwasher. The best method, however, seems to be microwaving. Wetting a sponge and putting it in the microwave for one to two minutes will kill more than 99 percent of the germs that could be hiding in there.

Of course, you could also try more disposable cleaning materials, which don't have the lifespan to build up too many pathogens. Regardless, if you haven't replaced your sponge or microwaved it in some time, be afraid. Or at least be more afraid of it than of the much cleaner items in your kitchen and bathroom.

Steam

I have just the thing for that cold . . .
Hot Steam

Another remedy you may hear about when you have a cold is to inhale hot steam. Whether sitting in the bathroom with a hot shower running or using a hot steam vaporizer, doctors and grandmothers alike advise that heated, humidified air will help cold sufferers. The idea is that hot steam will loosen up mucus in the nose or chest, enabling it to drain better, so that you can cough or blow it out. Some people also believe that the heat will kill any lingering cold viruses.

A comprehensive review looked at all the studies evaluating whether heated, humidified air helps with the common cold. In these studies, the heated steam is delivered to your nose through some sort of machine, whether through a mask (this seems to be popular in Britain) or through a vaporizer with a nozzle (the choice of most Americans). Since we should always ask ourselves what they did to convince a comparison group that they were getting the same treatment, you will be happy to know that the comparison groups in these studies usually received unheated humidified air.

Studies of hot steam for cold treatment from Israel and Britain did show some benefit for using hot steam in people with colds. People in these studies who received hot steam reported fewer cold symptoms in general, although no specific help was found for symptoms like cough or nasal congestion. However, three very good studies, all randomized controlled studies done in the United States, did not find any improvement in cold symptoms for people using hot steam. Neither their symptom scores, nor the cultures from their nose to see how many viruses were sticking around, were any better for those who used hot steam. Moreover, people using the steam did not think that it had helped.

These studies give a mixed picture as to whether hot steam will help your cold. With multiple good studies showing no difference and the overall mixed results, the experts conclude that hot steam is not recommended for treating cold symptoms.

Stress

Stress will make you sick

Stress works in the body in some interesting ways. When your body is under stress, it produces more of a hormone called cortisol that helps you think fast and brings more energy to your muscles, while slowing down the systems you do not need as much in the short term (such as your immune system or your digestive system). This is a great response in the short term. If you are running away from an animal that is about to attack you or you are rushing to beat a deadline, that stress response will give you the energy and focus you need. Stress can actually help you be more productive and manage challenges.

The problem for your body seems to come in when you are under stress for a long period of time. One example of a person under stress for a long time would be a parent taking care of a child with a chronic disease. Studies suggest that the white blood cells, the key cells of the body's immune system, seem to age more rapidly in parents of chronically ill children. People who are under stress for a long period do not make quite as much of a chemical called telomerase that helps to extend the life of your body's hardworking cells, and so their cells age more quickly. Depression works in the same way; people who are depressed for a long period of time also make less of this chemical that works to preserve the immune system's cells.

Whether it is because of the effect on these immune cells or by some other mechanism, stress seems to leave a person more susceptible to getting sick by germs to which they are exposed. A number of studies test this idea of stress making you sick by putting cold viruses directly into volunteers' noses and seeing who gets sick and who stays well. In a small study with seventeen subjects, their perceived stress and their overall mood were not connected to whether they got a cold; however, people who had had more major life events in the previous year were more likely to get colds. These included events that might be stressful, such as moving, graduating, marrying, or having someone close to them die. In a larger study of 394 volunteers, those with more psychological stress were more likely to get infected with the cold viruses put in their noses.

Stress might contribute to other kinds of sickness as well. There is some evidence that stress might make heart disease or headaches worse, even though stress does not cause a heart attack or headache or depression the way that a virus causes a cold. Chronic job stress can increase a person's overall risk of heart attacks by up to 50 percent, but the effect of stress varies from person to person. Depending on your genetics or on your perception of how much control you have in a particular situation, you might be less affected by stress. Some headaches, particularly tension headaches, are increased by stress, because some people increase muscle tension in their neck and shoulders when they are stressed. Stress has also been linked to slower healing of wounds and with flaring-up skin conditions such as herpes or acne (although it is sometimes difficult to tell which comes first—the acne or the stress). On the other hand, there is no evidence that stress causes cancer, diabetes, or many other diseases.

Stress is a complicated thing. How you handle it, what your underlying genetics are, and what other health problems you might have or be exposed to will alter how stress impacts your body and whether it will make you susceptible to various diseases.

Stress will give you high blood pressure

Stressful situations can raise your blood pressure temporarily. An increase in blood pressure is one of the ways your body responds to challenging situations that demand a flight-or-fight response. Much to our surprise, there is no evidence that stress causes high blood pressure over the long term. The evidence actually suggests that people with higher levels of stress do not have higher blood pressure overall. And there is no evidence that having lots of short-term spikes in your blood pressure raises your blood pressure over the long run.

While a few small studies that looked only at a few hundred people found connections between anxiety scores and long-term high blood pressure, other factors such as age, having parents with high blood pressure, or being obese were much more strongly tied to high blood pressure. While these studies already suggested that stress was not the most important issue in developing high blood pressure, their results were blown away by a huge study that suggested that stress levels might not play any role in developing high blood pressure over time. In a big study of 36,530 men and women who were followed for eleven years, they found no connection whatsoever between psychological stress scores for anxiety and depression and the development of high blood pressure. In fact, when they started this study, the people with higher levels of anxiety or depression symptoms actually had lower blood pressures than the people who had less psychological stress. As the eleven years of follow-up went on, the people who had increasing levels of anxiety and depression over time were even less likely to develop high blood pressure. This is the opposite of what you would expect. Instead of having more high blood pressure develop in the people who had increasing psychological distress, they actually had more cases of low blood pressure. These effects were not explained by the use of medicines for depression or high blood pressure, nor were they explained by differences in age, gender, baseline blood pressure, or other risk factors for developing high blood pressure.

Your family's genetics, how much fat you have around your middle, and other conditions like diabetes and high cholesterol are connected with the development of high blood pressure over the long term. People who are under stress may also do things that are less healthy for their hearts and for their blood pressure. Eating too much, drinking more alcohol, using recreational drugs, and not sleeping enough are all unhealthy behaviors that people do when they are feeling stressed. Even if stress itself is not causing long-term high blood pressure, these behaviors could put you at risk of not having a healthy heart or healthy blood pressure.

Just because stress is not the primary cause of high blood pressure, it does not mean that people with high blood pressure could not benefit from reducing their stress. If you suffer from high blood pressure, you should consider whether you do some of the unhealthy things just listed when you are under stress and whether you could eliminate or reduce them. Furthermore, certain behaviors that reduce your stress can also reduce your high blood pressure temporarily. Programs that teach meditation, progressive muscle relaxation, and other stress management programs have been shown to result in better blood pressure for some people struggling with high blood pressure.

Stress can give you a heart attack

As we have mentioned, your heart and other parts of your body respond to stressful situations in certain ways. A situation that causes anxiety, like having to speak in public or finding out very bad news, does make the beating of your heart speed up and make your blood pressure rise. Many people believe that stress of various kinds triggers heart attacks. For example, some people report that they think having a stressful job will lead to more heart attacks by increasing their blood pressure. Others believe that immediate stressful events, like hearing very shocking news, will trigger heart attacks directly. In a study of patients who had suffered from a heart attack, 15 to 30 percent of those who were admitted to a hospital had had a recent, severe emotionally stressful occurrence. While this points to a link between a heart attack and emotional stress, it is also possible that heart attack victims report more stressful events because they remember them clearly and assume that they are connected to their heart attacks. (This is that problem called recall bias again.)

So the bottom line is that stress can give you a heart attack— but it is important to realize that this is usually only a concern for people who already have a diseased heart. Stressful situations can reduce the amount of blood flowing to your heart as part of your body's short-term response to stress. If you already have partially blocked heart blood vessels or bad heart disease, it is possible that when a stressful situation increases your heart rate, increases your blood pressure, and causes less blood to flow to your heart, it could be enough to trigger a heart attack. This is not the cause of most heart attacks, but it is possible that this could happen. Again, having a heart attack during a stressful event requires that you have some sort of underlying problem with the blood vessels around your heart or problem in how your heart works. The diseases that affect the blood vessels around your heart and the heart itself are most often caused or made worse by having a high fat diet, not exercising, and smoking. Changing or avoiding these behaviors will go much further in preventing you from having a heart attack than trying to avoid any task or interaction that might cause you some stress.

Contrary to what many of us would expect, having short-term stressful reactions again and again is not clearly linked to developing heart disease over the long term. Scientists have found some evidence that both immediate stresses and having stress over a long time can lead to changes in how your immune system and your heart interact, and this can put you at more risk of having heart disease. Some studies also suggest that experiencing stress over time is tied to higher cholesterol and a greater chance of having a clogged artery. Once again, this might be because you react to stress by eating unhealthy things or not exercising—not because of the stress itself. But having high cholesterol and clogged arteries, along with other behaviors that are bad for your heart like smoking, puts you at much higher risk for heart disease and heart attacks. Other studies suggest that it is really not having enough rest and recovery time for your body, instead of the absolute level of stress, that puts you at increased risk for heart disease and heart attacks over the long term.

There clearly are ways in which excess stress could have a negative effect on your heart. The biggest lesson you should take from this is that there are important ways you can manage your stress and protect your heart at the same time. You can never avoid stress altogether. Exercising, eating a diet that is higher in fruits and vegetables and lower in fats, and quitting smoking are probably the very best things you can do for your heart in the long term. Exercising, in particular, will keep your heart healthy and will help you have less stress at the same time.

Stretching

You should stretch before you exercise

Almost anyone who works out, plays sports, runs, or engages in regular exercise will tell you that you should absolutely stretch first. Stretching is supposed to help you perform better. Even more importantly, stretching is supposed to prevent injuries. The idea of not stretching before a run or before a game is anathema to most athletes. Entire books are devoted to describing the best ways to stretch, and careers of coaches and trainers have been built upon their knowledge of proper stretching. How could we even suggest something so dangerous as not stretching before exercise?

As much as it may shock you, there is good scientific evidence that stretching does not reduce your chance of being injured during sports or exercise. Several meta-analyses or comprehensive reviews have been done to compile all of the studies on this subject. In a 2004 systematic review by scientists at the Centers for Disease Control, the authors reviewed 361 studies and identified six that most rigorously tested whether stretching reduced the chance of getting injured. Most of these studies tested the effects of stretching for people going through basic training in the military or for high school and college football players. The combined verdict from these studies was that the enhanced flexibility created through stretching did not reduce the injuries seen in sporting or fitness activities. So even if you stretched carefully, you were still just as likely to get a pulled muscle as a person who did not stretch first.

Even if stretching will not help you prevent injuries, you still may cling to your stretching routine because you think it prevents your muscles from getting sore. In particular, many people stretch before or after exercise or at both times in order to prevent their muscles from being sore the day after they exercise. Another excellent systematic review compiled the results of ten randomized trials that looked at the effect of stretching before or after physical activity on muscle soreness. These were not great studies—they were small and of questionable quality—but they do give us some idea of what stretching does for muscle soreness. And the answer is: very little! Stretching had very little to no effect whatsoever on muscle soreness in half a day to three days after the physical activity.

There is also evidence that stretching has some negative effects. Stretching does improve your flexibility, but this is not always a good thing. Instead of improving your performance, stretching has been associated with temporary deficits or decreases in your strength, with increased blood pressure, with worse jumping performance, and with worse flexing strength of your ankles. These is also some suggestion that people who are more flexible do not run as well, but these results are mixed.

Let's summarize the research: Stretching does not prevent injuries. Stretching does not keep your muscles from getting sore later on. Stretching can actually make you perform worse. This seems like craziness! Rachel can hear the gasps of horror and disbelief from her fellow runners (most of whom are much faster than she is and who also spend a lot of time stretching). And yet study after study tells us that you are not going to get any benefit out of stretching before you run. One of the most recent studies, done by the USA Track and Field organization, looked at about 1,400 runners who were randomly assigned to stretch or not stretch before their runs. Even this pro-running organization found that stretching did not prevent running injuries.

What about warming up? Studies of warming up look at activities other than stretching, such as walking, running, or calisthenics, that are done before a more vigorous athletic activity. The evidence on warming up is not as clear. While study after study tells us that stretching before exercise does not prevent injuries, some of the studies of other forms of warming up before exercise show that this practice will reduce injuries. In a systematic review compiling all the randomized, controlled studies (i.e., the good studies) of warming up before exercise, three of the studies showed that warming up first did reduce injuries later. The other two studies did not find any effect from warming up. The conclusion was that there is not sufficient evidence to say whether a routine warm-up before your exercise will help you prevent injuries, but there is some suggestion that this might work.

Continue those warm-ups if you must (although we'll have to keep compiling the studies on whether or not that really works), but stretching is not going to help you be a better or safer runner!

Eating sugar causes diabetes

Many people know that diabetes is a sugar problem, and that people with diabetes cannot have too much sugar. Along those lines, many people believe that eating sugar causes diabetes. They blame diabetes on having a chronic sweet tooth or on not being able to resist a sugary diet.

In order to understand diabetes, it is helpful to have an idea of what your body does with sugar. Your body gets much of its energy by converting the sugar and carbohydrates you eat into a special form of sugar called glucose. Glucose is the sugar that most of your body needs to operate. In order to absorb glucose, your body manufactures a special hormone called insulin that regulates the amount of glucose in your blood and the amount that is absorbed into different parts of the body. Your pancreas makes this insulin, and without insulin, you cannot absorb glucose into your body's cells. If you do not have enough insulin or if your body does not respond to insulin, you cannot absorb or use sugar in the way your body needs.

There are two types of diabetes, called type 1 diabetes and type 2 diabetes. Type 1 diabetes usually develops in younger people, typically in children, when the pancreas stops making the insulin your body needs in order to absorb sugar. How much sugar you eat has absolutely nothing to do with developing type 1 diabetes. It is caused by genetics and other factors that trigger the pancreas to stop working normally. Type 2 diabetes usually develops in adults, although it sometimes develops in children as well. In type 2 diabetes, your body becomes resistant to the effects of insulin, so your body does not absorb sugar in the ways it is supposed to. Type 2 diabetes is caused by both genetic factors and lifestyle factors. In particular, being overweight significantly increases your risk of developing type 2 diabetes. It is possible that you could be overweight from eating too much sugar, but you could also be overweight from eating too much fat or any other diet high in calories. While eating a lot of sugar can certainly make your diet very high in calories, the sugar does not directly cause the diabetes.

Several studies in large groups of people have found that those who drink more sugar-sweetened beverages have higher rates of diabetes and more cases of type 2 diabetes. While this suggests a connection between sugar and diabetes, it is the connection that occurs because sugary drinks make you gain weight. In a systematic review that compiled studies looking at sugar-sweetened beverages and weight gain, the researchers found that drinking more sweet beverages was connected to more obesity and to being overweight for children and adults. Taking in sugar is not independently connected to developing diabetes; obesity is what is really connected to developing diabetes.

People with diabetes do not need to stay away from sugar altogether. They can eat sweets or starches, but they should eat them in moderation, as part of a healthy meal plan. Having a healthy diet means eating plenty of fruits and vegetables, some meats or proteins, and not more than a few servings of foods containing carbohydrates.

Even if you are not diabetic or if you now understand that sugar will not give you diabetes, there are plenty of reasons to eat sugar in moderation. Gaining too much weight or developing lots of cavities are bad effects from a diet too full of sugar. However, you do not need to worry that diabetes will automatically follow from your sweet tooth.

Television

Sitting too close to the TV will ruin your eyes

D on't sit so close to the television! It will ruin your eyesight!" Many a child has heard this admonishment when staring at the TV or peering intently at a computer screen. Aaron watches more television than most people (despite being a highly productive researcher and professor), and he is blind as a bat without his glasses. Is his television-watching to blame for his nearsightedness?

This is one of those myths that we cannot disprove definitively because no one has done a great big study where some children are forced to watch television up close for hours and hours. (And no one is going to do that study.) We can tell you that there is absolutely no evidence that sitting close to the television or computer screen ruins your eyesight. Whether you sit within inches of the screen or whether you watch for hours and hours, there is no evidence that television will ruin your eyes.

This myth may have come from the early days of television. The first television sets actually emitted a lot of radiation. In fact, these televisions put out more than 100,000 times the radiation that the federal health officials deem safe. Sitting really close to those old televisions in the 1950s might have been a risk for a person's eyes. But this radiation from televisions is not a risk anymore. Televisions have improved in so many ways since then, and they no longer emit lots of radiation.

The reason this myth may stick around is because sitting close to the television can give you eye strain. When you sit close to the television, when you stare at a screen for a long period of time, or when you read in the dark, you do strain your eyes. Eye strain can cause eye pain, make your eyes dry and your vision fuzzy, and can even give you a headache. Thankfully, eye strain is a temporary condition. When you stop watching television or when you move into better conditions, your vision returns to normal. Just like running may give you tired legs but does not weaken your leg muscles permanently, most eye strain does not ruin your eyes forever. When you rest your eyes, they return to normal.

It is important to note that there may be a different kind of connection between a child who sits close to the television and a child with bad vision. When children need glasses, they will often start to sit closer and closer to the television or other screens, blackboards, or books. This is not because the television is ruining their eyes, but because they need help seeing! Children should have their vision tested regularly, and parents should be even more quick to get this testing for a child who seems to be sitting closer and closer to the television.

As pediatricians, we feel obligated to remind parents that there are other reasons why it might be a good idea to limit how much television a child watches. Even if their eyes are perfectly safe, watching too much television is connected with children being overweight or obese. Television might be particularly bad for babies and young children. Watching television, even educational videos or programs designed for babies and toddlers, has been associated with delayed learning and development. The American Academy of Pediatrics recommends that children under the age of two years not watch any television at all, and that television watching be limited to less than two hours per day for older children. Your mother was wrong about television hurting your eyes, but she may have been right on track about it hurting your developing brain.

Toilet Seats

Touching a toilet seat will make you sick

Despite the fears of countless parents, no reputable health organization has ever targeted toilets as a serious way to catch an infection. It's important to remember that most serious viruses and bacteria can't live for very long outside the body. They are no more likely to survive on a toilet than on any other household surface. Let's face it. Most of you are really concerned about picking up a really bad disease from the toilet. So let us put your mind at ease. You can't catch HIV from a toilet. Nor are you likely to catch a sexually transmitted disease from a toilet (see our next toilet seat myth for more information about that). You're pretty much safe from parasites as well. That's not how those are spread.

You also need to remember that most infections do not enter through intact skin. They need to get into the mouth, an open wound, or a mucus membrane. So even if you sat on a germ, it wouldn't necessarily infect you. If you wash your hands, anything you touched should be taken care of. Again, toilets pose no special danger.

Studies indicate that hardier viruses, like influenza A, can be found on toilets in day care centers. But viruses can be found even more commonly on kitchen dishcloths and diaper-changing areas. Toilets aren't special.

In fact, there are lots of other things that are likely far more infectious than the toilet, and we bet you don't think about them at all. Do you know how dirty money can be? Think about how many people have touched that. How about the phone? Your keyboard? In fact, people who eat at their work desks are far more likely to get infected than those who touch the toilet.

Of course, we will still flush it with our feet when we can. Come on.

You can get gonorrhea from the toilet seat

In an episode of one of our favorite television shows, *Seinfeld*, one of Jerry's girlfriends has a mysterious "tractor story" that she is reluctant to tell him until their relationship progresses. Jerry thinks the story is going to explain the mysterious scar on the girl's leg, but instead, the story ends up being that she supposedly got gonorrhea from sitting on the seat of a tractor in her bathing suit (at least, that is what her boyfriend told her was the cause).

While relatively few people spend time on tractor seats, a lot of people believe that they might get a sexually transmitted disease from a toilet seat. The fear of toilet seats springs from the idea that public toilets are filthy places full of bacteria, but also because many have heard that toilet seats could be to blame for such an infection. It seems a lot easier to blame the toilet than to blame your boyfriend.

When we refer to sexually transmitted diseases, we are talking about infections caused by either bacteria or viruses that are typically passed only when one person has sex or contact with the sexual organs of another person. These are diseases like chlamydia, gonorrhea, herpes, and infection with HIV. The scary idea that you could get one of these serious infections from a toilet seat is enough to make anyone want to hover over the toilet bowl, but it also offers an excuse for how you may have gotten one of these infections without sex being involved.

There is no research proving that people get infected with

sexually transmitted diseases from sitting on toilet seats. This does not mean that it is impossible to get infected from a toilet seat, but there is no evidence either way. There are a few published cases where physicians describe patients who they believe may have become infected after direct contact with exceptionally dirty toilet seats, but in these cases, they cannot prove that the patients did not have physical or sexual contact of some kind with a person who was infected. The majority of experts, including the president of the American Society for Microbiology, report never seeing or hearing about cases of people actually acquiring an STD from a toilet seat (unless they were having sex with another person while on the toilet)!

Even though it may be theoretically possible to get infected from a toilet seat, there are many reasons why this is very unlikely to happen. First of all, most of the bugs that cause sexually transmitted diseases in humans do not survive well outside the human body. The viruses that cause herpes and AIDS do not live outside of the body for long. They dry out and die when exposed to air, and there have been no próven cases of people getting herpes or AIDS from a toilet seat. The bacteria that cause infections like chlamydia and gonorrhea do not live much longer. Second, for these bacteria to get onto the toilet seat, someone would first need to leave their bodily fluids on the toilet seat. Obviously, public toilet seats do end up with a lot of urine on them, but urine is not where these germs live. These germs live in the fluids in your vagina or penis, or sometimes in your blood. It is much less likely that someone would be rubbing against a toilet seat or sitting in a way that would leave discharge or secretions from their vagina or penis on the seat. People also do not usually bleed onto the toilet seat. Even if the bug did get onto the seat in one of these secretions and did manage to survive, it is not a sure thing that someone coming into contact with that bug-infested fluid would become infected. In fact, it is quite unlikely. The bugs would have to be transferred from the seat into your urethra or to your genital tract, or maybe into a cut or sore somewhere on your private parts. You would need to touch the gunk on the toilet seat with one of these parts. Finally, even if someone did leave a germ, it survived, and you touched it, it very well might not be enough of the germs to cause you an infection. For many of these infections, you need to come in contact with a pretty large number of them to make you sick. It is theroetically possible that just one or two germs might infect you, but it is incredibly unlikely.

If you know much about the different types of sexually transmitted infections, you might be wondering about the possibility of getting crabs or scabies from a toilet seat. Crabs are lice that live in your pubic hair. They are a different type of lice than the lice that live in the hair on your head, but they cause lots of itching and irritation. Just like the lice that live in the hair on your head, pubic lice are very contagious. Crabs or pubic lice are probably the infection that you could get the most easily from a toilet seat. This has not been studied well, and it would be very, very rare, but it is possible that you could get crabs from a toilet seat. Pubic lice can live for about twenty-four hours outside of the body, so they would not live there very long, but it is possible that one might wait on a toilet seat to infect you. Again, this is very unlikely, but the experts say it is possible.

Scabies is somewhat similar to crabs in that it is an itchy skin disease caused by little bugs called mites. Scabies can be spread through sexual contact or through being skin-to-skin or very close to someone with scabies. Experts also say that it might be possible to contract scabies if the mites are left on the toilet seat. This is, again, very unlikely, as things like close hugging or handshaking are only very rarely a way that people get infected with scabies. Scabies can live outside the body longer than some other bugs, but they still only live for about twenty-four to thirty-six hours outside of the human body.

Toilet seats are pretty gross (though they may be cleaner than sponges and faucets), but your risk of getting any sort of infection from a toilet seat, let alone a sexually transmitted infection, is incredibly low. You would be much, much better off using a condom regularly with your partners than worrying obsessively about the toilet seat. Not having sex is also a much more effective way to avoid sexually transmitted diseases than avoiding public toilets. While it might be reasonable to clean off the toilet seat with a wad of toilet paper or to try to squat without touching one, the most important advice is to wash your hands after using the bathroom and practice safe sex.

Vaccines

You shouldn't get a vaccine if you are sick

We can't tell you how many times we've been asked about this in the office. Most people understand why it's important to get vaccinated, but there are a lot of misunderstandings about when or how to get vaccines. One of these misunderstandings is that vaccines don't work, or are even dangerous, if you are ill.

First, it is worth reviewing how vaccines work. In a nutshell, vaccines contain substances that mimic the germs that can cause certain illnesses. While the substances in vaccines cannot cause actual illness, they cause the body's immune system to react in such a way as to create antibodies that can later defeat the actual illness.

As with many of the myths in this book, there is a kernel of truth in the myth that has run amok. In this case, there is some evidence that vaccines could cause changes in how your body reacts to particular things, like the TB skin test. This led some to theorize that vaccines would lead to increased illnesses in the period after they were given. Some parents worry that if the body is busy responding to the vaccine, it will not be able to respond to other things that might make you sick. Fortunately, that's not so. A study of almost 500 children in Germany found that infants in the first three months of life who received vaccines had fewer, not more, illnesses from germs both related and not related to the vaccines. Another study of children in

Alaska receiving the DTP (diphtheria, tetanus, pertussis) vaccine found no relationship between getting vaccines and increased risks of other infections.

Another strain of this myth centers on the idea that vaccines won't work as well if you are sick. That's not true, either. A study in Canada found that having an upper respiratory tract infection in the month before a vaccination, during a vaccination, or up to a week after a vaccination had no effect on the body's response to the vaccine. A different study in Haiti a decade earlier also found that neither malnutrition nor acute infections affected the vaccine response. One more study from the mid-1990s in Atlanta found that the success of the vaccine in achieving the proper response was nearly identical between well children and those with upper respiratory infections, mild fevers, ear infections, diarrhea, and mild illnesses. Nor were there any more adverse events in the ill children than in the well children. Vaccines work just as well when you are sick with most illnesses. This myth is of concern because parents who delay getting vaccines for their children because of a mild illness may not return promptly to catch up on the shots. And children who fall behind, or do not receive their vaccines, are at increased risk to get vaccine-preventable illnesses. We need to use every opportunity to give vaccines in order to optimally protect babies and children from these diseases.

The big groups that make recommendations on vaccines, like the Centers for Disease Control and the American Academy of Pediatrics, recommend that people who are severely, and sometimes moderately, ill delay vaccines until they are better. Your doctor can help you in these kinds of decisions. But there's nothing to fear from getting vaccines when your child is mildly ill. They don't increase the risk to your child (and may even reduce it) and the vaccines will work just fine.

Getting the flu vaccine is more important for adults than children

As pediatricians, this one hits closer to home than some of the other myths. It's hard enough convincing people that the flu shot is important for the elderly. It's even harder to convince parents that it's important for their children.

Look, we acknowledge how hard it is to get your children vaccinated. They are getting so many shots already, and you don't want to add one more. It can be hard to get an appointment, especially during flu season, when everyone else is trying to get their children the shot. There are often shortages, making it time-consuming even to know whether it is worth going for the shot. And then, even if everything works out and you can fit them in, you need to take off work or rearrange appointments or have your child miss school. Is the flu shot really that important?

People also question the value of the flu shot for children because of a general perception that children aren't really at risk from the flu. You may have read the chapter about how influenza kills many people each year, but those people are mostly the elderly, right?

The short answer to that question used to be yes. Until recently, more than 90 percent of deaths that occurred from flu in the United States were in people sixty-five years old or older. Nonetheless, the regular flu still kills and hospitalizes children and babies every year. With the introduction of H1N1, the picture for children becomes more of a concern. Here are some facts from the outbreak in 2009–2010:

> The cumulative hospitalization rate for flu for children up to four years of age was 8.3 per 10,000. This was two to three times higher than the rates for adults, and still more than twice the hospitalization rate for people over sixty-five.

There were 279 lab-confirmed flu deaths, which was four times the average of the previous five years.
Of those 279 deaths, 226 were from the H1N1 strain.

No matter how you want to look at it, H1N1 has changed the game. Kids are more at risk than ever. They are more likely to be hospitalized, and more likely to die. So if you want to protect your kids, you need to get them the shot.

So far, this argument ignores the larger truth about vaccines. Sometimes we don't get vaccinated to protect ourselves. We often get vaccinated to protect others. It's a societal good.

The reason we vaccinate health care workers is to protect patients just as much as the clinicians. Sometimes, the reason we vaccinate older children is to protect younger children in the house. And we vaccinate the general population in part to protect the elderly. When we come in contact with older people vaccination makes it much less likely we will pass the disease on to them. Many children have regular contact with their grandparents. If children are ill, even if they are not at risk themselves, they can be a risk to the elderly. It's not an argument used often, but that makes it no less true. It's important to vaccinate children not only to protect them, but also to protect those that they love.

Too many vaccines will weaken your immune system

Shots are no fun. And, believe us, doctors and nurses don't like giving them any more than you like getting them. People are always looking for reasons not to get shots. This myth is one of the most commonly used excuses. Parents worry about the number of shots their babies are supposed to get and will often develop elaborate plans to spread the shots out over a much longer period of time so that the immune system does not need to respond to too many shots at once.

Let's start by recognizing that the human body has an enormous capacity to respond to potential threats. You are constantly exposed to foreign substances that stimulate your immune system. In a manuscript specifically designed to answer this question in the journal *Pediatrics*, Dr. Paul Offit and colleagues estimated that infants have the capacity to respond to about 10,000 vaccines at any one time. No vaccine could "use up" the immune system. In fact, estimates showed that if a child received eleven vaccines at one time, that might occupy about 0.1 percent of the immune system. You'd never notice that.

Moreover, this argument against vaccines assumes that the cells being occupied or destroyed in the vaccine response process are not replaced. You body is constantly making new cells, though, so this never occurs.

Another point, often overlooked, is that it is not the number of vaccines, or even the number of shots, that matters. It's the number of antigens in those vaccines. An antigen is a molecule that the immune system recognizes. The immune system decides whether any molecules it comes in contact with belong to itself or whether they should be treated as foreign intruders. Vaccines are specifically designed to show the immune system an antigen that belongs to a particular disease so that the immune system will be armed and equipped to fight against that disease if it sees it again. Advances in technology have helped scientists create vaccines that contain fewer and fewer antigens and yet achieve a good response from your immune system. Back in the day, a single smallpox vaccine had over 200 different proteins in it. In the 1980s, the seven vaccines routinely given to children contained more than 2,000 antigens. Now the eleven vaccines in the currently recommended schedule have only about 125 antigens in all. Even though it seems like a lot of shots, the immune system has to do far less work to respond to the current set of antigens than children's immune systems had had to do the past thirty years.

Don't take our word for it. Research has shown that giving vaccines alone or in combination does not affect their ability to achieve a response. A trial comparing the effectiveness of the MMR (measles, mumps, rubella) and chickenpox vaccines given together and alone showed no difference in their effectiveness. The immune system responds how it should whether the shots are given separately or at the same time. Another study compared the effect of giving MMR, DTP, and polio boosters at the same time to giving the vaccines individually, one after the other. The vaccines were just as effective when they were given at the same time as when they were given individually. The immune system responded just as well when the shots were combined together. The same result was seen when looking at adding hepatitis B vaccine to other vaccines in infants. Your body can easily handle the load.

If you remain concerned that giving a vaccine weakens the immune system, studies show us this is not the case. Remember that study of almost 500 children in Germany? They had fewer illnesses after the vaccines, not more. The babies' immune systems were working fine! In fact, the immune systems in the children getting the shots may have even been working better. There was also that study of children in Alaska receiving the DTP vaccine where children who got that vaccine did not get more infections from other sources.

Some have theorized that giving more vaccines over time has led to an increase in conditions like autism. We addressed that myth in our first book, *Don't Swallow Your Gum!*, and two years later, there is still no good evidence to support that theory. One huge study after another concludes that there is no link between vaccines and autism. Those ideas also ignore the truths revealed here—that the number of antigens children are exposed to has been going down, not up.

We don't want to poke your children any more than you do. But they really do benefit from those vaccines.

Vitamin C

I have just the thing for that cold . . . Vitamin C

Claiming vitamin C is useless for colds is enough to get one beaten up in some circles. If Aaron did not have ninja skills, we would never get out of auditoriums alive when we dispel this myth. Vitamin C is on every health food and pharmacy shelf, and people take it both to prevent colds and to treat them. Just because many people use something faithfully and swear by it does not mean that it works.

Tests of whether vitamin C prevents colds have been done on thousands of people. The research investigating vitamin C is impressive. When scientists combine the results of twenty-three studies investigating whether vitamin C prevents colds in normal people, there is no significant improvement. Vitamin C does not prevent you from getting a cold. In studies involving over 11,000 people taking 200 mg or more of vitamin C a day, the vitamin C did not prevent colds. In a subset of people studied, vitamin C came a little closer to looking like it would work (although the results were still statistically insignificant). In people who engaged in extreme exercise in extreme conditions—marathon runners, soldiers training in the Arctic, and skiers—vitamin C almost looked like it worked to prevent colds. But it still made no significant difference. If you plan on engaging in seriously strenuous exercise in very cold conditions, you might consider taking a vitamin C supplement in the hope that it just might work, but otherwise there is no evidence to justify taking regular doses.

Sadly, vitamin C does not kill the viruses that cause colds, nor does it seem to make your cold symptoms better. In seven studies looking at the treatment of the common cold, scientists found no improvement in symptoms if you took vitamin C. It was no better than a placebo; neither one improved the cold symptoms. Based on the results of eleven studies of more than 6,000 people, taking vitamin C does not make the duration of your cold any shorter or your cold any less severe. In these trials, people took doses up to 4 grams (4,000 mg) and did not see a benefit in cold symptoms. Vitamin C doesn't work!

Vitamin E

Vitamin E helps scars heal

Vitamin E has become a popular remedy to apply to cuts, scrapes, and even surgical wounds to help scars heal. Some people believe it will take your scar away or get rid of those ugly stretch marks. Many health professionals, including doctors, nurses, and medical students, recommend vitamin E to their patients to improve the look of their scars.

In the lab, vitamin E has been found to have an antioxidant effect, but there is no good scientific evidence that vitamin E actually does anything to improve how a wound heals. At first glance, the evidence looks promising. In one study of eighty patients with very large scars, or keloids, putting a silicone sheet that contained vitamin E overnight on the scar seemed to improve the appearance of scars more than using silicone sheets that did not have vitamin E.

Unfortunately, other studies have not found similarly good effects when using vitamin E. In a study of patients who had skin cancers removed, each patient was given two ointments to put on either end of the wound. One ointment was a pure moisturizer called Aquaphor, and the other was Aquaphor mixed with vitamin E. Neither the patients nor the physicians knew which ointment was being put where on the scar. Neither patients, physicians, nor an independent reviewer could see any benefit from the vitamin E ointment at one, four, or twelve weeks after the surgery. For 90 percent of the patients, the patients, physicians, and reviewers thought the vitamin E–treated area of the scar looked the same or even worse. A third of patients also developed a contact dermatitis, which is an itchy rash, from the vitamin E. Another group of researchers studied 159 patients who had surgery to remove contractures, or tightening of the skin, that was produced after having been burned. After these patients had surgery, they were randomized to either put a vitamin E ointment on the wound, a steroid ointment, or a plain moisturizer. Neither the vitamin E nor the steroid made any difference in the thickness or size of the scar or the overall cosmetic appearance. The results from these studies suggest that the limited evidence in favor of vitamin E is questionable. In two careful studies, the researchers could not find a healing effect from vitamin E, and it even caused rashes or side effects in some patients. We have said this before about other treatments, but if something does not work and seems to have a good chance of making a problem worse or giving you another side effect, it makes sense to stay away from that "treatment."

Vitamin E does not seem to be a good answer for scar-healing, but you might actually think about onions. Really. An extract from onions has been shown in randomized trials to improve the texture and redness of scars in patients, as well as to have good effects on the cells involved with scar formation in the laboratory. Gels such as Mederma contain this onion extract. More research into what might work to really help wound-healing or to get rid of our scars or stretch marks would be very welcome.

Warts

You will get warts from handling frogs or toads

No one likes warts, and frogs and toads aren't very popular either, so it's no wonder they are linked. Moreover, many toads and frogs have bumps and such on their bodies that look like warts. These protrusions often seem to ooze disgusting liquid as well, lending credence to the idea that they must be infectious in some way. The next conclusion is that they could give you those bumps or warts.

One part of this is true. Warts are contagious. Warts are actually caused by an infection, by viruses in fact. One virus in specific, human papillomavirus (HPV), is responsible for warts. There are many types of HPV and it is such a common virus that three quarters of people will get a wart at some time.

In fact, one strain of human papillomavirus even causes genital warts. This virus has been in the news more in the last few years because it is linked to cervical cancer in women. There is now a vaccine for the human papillomavirus that causes genital warts in order to try to prevent cervical cancer in women. We assume, and hope, that no one thinks they caught those kinds of warts from a frog or toad.

Warts of any kind are not easy to get rid of. Because they are caused by a virus, it's actually possible for them to spread or re-infect you. Treatment with salicylic acid tries to burn off the warts chemically. This treatment can take weeks and sometimes hurts. Some doctors will freeze warts with liquid nitrogen, but that's not painless either. Newer therapies involve the use of blister beetle extract or lasers. None of these is fun, and they don't always work right away.

Regardless, the truth is you can't catch any type of warts from an amphibian and that is for the simple reason that there is no human papillomavirus on them. Those bumps and protrusions that look like warts are actually defense mechanisms for the frogs or toads. That stuff the frogs and toads ooze is often poison, and it's so nasty that animals have been known to spit the frogs or toads out almost immediately after putting them in their mouths.

So yes, frogs and toads are yucky. Yes, they look like they have warts on their skin. And yes, you can "catch" warts in the sense that they are caused by a viral infection. But you can't get warts from a toad or frog. That's a myth.

Wet Hair

Going outside with wet hair will make you sick

Rachel has had long hair most of her life. Sometimes, it's tempting not to dry all that hair, but she knows very well the looks of horror and the gasps of concern that will greet her if she heads out of the house without drying her long locks. Especially in the colder months, going outside with wet hair is considered a clear recipe for bringing on a cold or pneumonia or other health disaster. In a survey of parents bringing their children in to the emergency department because they had a cold, 41 percent of the parents believed that going out with wet hair in cold weather could cause a cold. But what's the truth here? If you are too lazy or running too late to dry your hair, are you putting your health at risk?

The first thing to consider in answering these questions is just what it is that makes you sick. Having wet hair does not make you sick. Being cold or getting chilled because you have wet hair does not make you sick. It's not even the combination of cold weather and wet hair that makes you sick. What makes you sick is when your body is infected with a virus or with bacteria. Developing a cold is the type of sickness that most people worry about when they go out with wet hair. If you learn one thing from this book, it should be that colds are caused by viruses, most often by viruses from the rhinovirus family. Without a virus sneaking into your nose or mouth or other wet parts, you are not going to get sick. You get sick because someone who is infected with a rhinovirus sneezes or coughs, sending tiny droplets of fluid and rhinovirus into the air around you or onto their hands or onto something else you might come in contact with. When you breathe in that air full of tiny virus-filled drops of fluid or when you shake their cough-contaminated hand, you get some of that virus into your nose or mouth. It's that virus that makes you sick—not your wet hair!

The next question might be whether your wet hair makes you more likely to be infected by those viruses that cause our coughs and colds. Having wet hair does make you feel cooler, especially when the temperatures are low. Does that extra chill make you more susceptible to getting a cold? The science suggests that this is not the case. In study after study, scientists have tested this question by putting the viruses that cause colds directly into volunteers' noses and then making them spend time in different kinds of conditions. They make some of the volunteers stay in chilled rooms or freezing conditions, while others are in warmer rooms. And they make some of the volunteers have wet hair, while others have dry hair. In these studies, volunteers exposed to the cold-causing viruses are no more likely to get infected by those viruses if they have wet hair or if they have dry hair. Whether or not they get cold or are in cold conditions doesn't make any difference either. Getting chilled, whether from your hair or from the cold weather, does not make you susceptible to getting infected with a cold virus. There is no scientific evidence that getting cold will cause your cold.

For those of you who are still not convinced, there may be one piece of evidence in your favor. There was a study where people who had their feet chilled were more likely to report cold symptoms. Does this mean that you might notice more cold symptoms if your feet are cold than if your head is chilled from your wet hair? Maybe. That study has not been done. But, even here, the important thing to remember is that there is still no support for the chilled feet causing the cold symptoms. You may just notice your symptoms more because you have cold feet. Some exports hypothesize that having a very cold part of the body causes a reflex in which you have less blood flow to your nose and upper airways, and that this somehow inhibits your body's defenses, converting a viral infection that you didn't really notice into one that is causing you symptoms like a stuffy nose. But this hypothesis has never been proven. It's just as likely that when you have had really cold feet from your wet boots or a really cold head from your wet hair, you get worried about whether you are going to get sick and so you notice your sniffles right away.

The next time your mother scolds you about your wet hair, you can explain about the rhinoviruses that cause colds and the volunteers who spent all that time in the cold with wet hair and viruses stuck in their noses. Or, you can just run out the door really fast!

Wounds

You should uncover a wound at night to let it air out and heal

Most children wound themselves at one point or another. (Even though cautious parents are tempted to keep their children in a protective cocoon, most of us cannot maintain the bubble.) When we hurt ourselves at any age, we often hear the advice to expose the cut to the air so that it can heal better.

Most people who believe in this time-honored tradition do so for any number of reasons. Some believe that airing out a wound reduces the likelihood of infection. Others believe that drying the wound allows it to scab and will make the wound heal faster. Many also think there is something special about air, and letting the air get to the wound is a good thing.

This is completely backward.

When you cut yourself or sustain a wound, your skin heals itself by growing new cells out from the edges toward each other. These cells actually need a moist environment in which to grow and spread. In fact, when the wound dries out, or a hard scab forms, it can become more difficult for these cells to get where they need to be. Not only that, but a hard scab can permanently force these cells into undesirable formations, thus resulting in scars.

Ironically, wounds need exactly what many people have been claiming was harmful. A moist, covered environment is best. There have been a number of studies showing this is true. A study published in the *Journal of Surgical Research* in 1991 described ninety-two wounds inflicted on four piglets. These wounds were treated with eight different dressing regimens. Contrary to what many thought, they found that inert or dry bandages, such as dry gauze, caused wounds to take longer to heal. Another study in the *Annals of Plastic Surgery* in 1995 compared wet, moist, and dry gauze dressings on pig wounds. They found that wet, bandaged wounds healed two days faster than dry ones, and one day faster than moist ones. The moist or wet bandages also led to less necrosis (necrosis is a bad thing where your tissues die) and better quality of healing.

And if you aren't convinced by pigs (although they seem to be the animal of choice for wound studies because their skin is most like ours), a study was conducted in twenty humans and published in 2008. These subjects allowed themselves to receive abrasions and were then given different types of bandages or no bandages. Wound-healing was checked on days 1, 3, 5, 7, 10, and 14 and judged on contraction, color, and luminance. These people took wound-healing seriously. They found that every kind of occlusive dressing (that means a dressing that covers up the wound tightly) performed better than no dressing at all. Anything that covers up the wound is better than leaving it open!

Additionally, no study has found that using dressings increases the rate of infection. There's no truth to the idea that drying out the wound is better in terms of infection.

So while your mother (or grandmother) may tell you it's a good idea to air out that cut or let it dry out, there is a wealth of evidence showing you should do the opposite. You should cover wounds, and not allow them to dry completely, as this will lead to faster and better healing with no increase in infection.

You should lick a wound or put a cut finger in your mouth

You know you've done it. You cut your finger or some other part of your body, and your first impulse was to put it in your mouth.

Maybe you've licked a wound. Maybe you've sucked on a cut until it stopped bleeding. It seemed natural; you've seen lots of animals do it. But think about it. Is that really a good idea?

There are reasons that animals do this. Sometimes, licking a wound is the best way for a wild animal to clean it. But come on, we humans have a few better options. (Water, in particular, comes to mind.) There is also a body of research that shows there are compounds in saliva that might aid healing. But even those papers don't come to the conclusion that you should lick a wound. Instead, they end by discussing how they will try and isolate those compounds to create new creams or medicine.

Why shouldn't you use your mouth? The mouth is not especially clean. If you read our previous book, this should come as no surprise. The human mouth is full of bacteria, and licking a cut is a great way to get those germs into your cut. For example, the *New England Journal of Medicine* reported on a German man with diabetes who licked his thumb after a bicycle accident. Although the wound was minor, his thumb became infected with *Eikenella corrodens*, and it had to be amputated. That bacterium is commonly found in the mouth, and it was believed that his licking the wound led to the loss of his thumb.

Another report linked a rare circumcision ritual with genital herpes. A small number of Orthodox Jews practice circumcision in which the man performing the circumcision sucks the blood from the baby's wound until it stops bleeding. A manuscript published in *Pediatrics* described a number of Jewish infants who developed genital herpes not long after birth. Many of them had pretty severe infections or complications. When the available infants were tested, all were positive for carrying herpes in their mouths.

Although these are extreme examples, your mouths are not clean. You wouldn't clean a wound with a dirty wet rag, so don't clean one with your dirty wet mouth. Keep your tongue, and your mouth, away from cuts and wounds.

Zinc

I have just the thing for that cold . . . Zinc

It seems like we have gone through a hundred potential cures for the common cold, and yet nothing seems to work. Here is a scintillating surprise: zinc might, just might help you with your sniffles and stuffiness.

When we first considered the evidence for zinc and colds, using a review that combined the results from eight different studies, zinc did not seem to prevent or shorten colds. A newer review published in 2011 includes almost twice as many studies, and the combined new evidence suggests that zinc could actually improve your cold symptoms and shorten their duration by about a day. The effect is strongest if you start taking zinc within the first twenty-four hours that you experience cold symptoms. Those zealous people rushing to offer you a zinc lozenge may have a point; zinc works best if you use it at the very first sniffle!

Whether zinc can actually prevent you from developing a cold remains an open question. The review provided some evidence that people who took zinc regularly for at least five months (that's a long-term commitment!) had fewer colds, but these studies were of lower quality than the studies looking at the impact of zinc on cold symptoms. The research quality is such that this will need to be studied more before we have a definitive answer as to whether zinc really prevents colds.

On balance, it is important to know that using those zinc lozenges could also make you feel bad in new ways. Zinc tastes horrible! In a blind taste test, we bet it would come in third after a rotting dead skunk and old gym socks. In fact, zinc lozenges were more likely to make people feel nauseous than they were to improve cold symptoms. People who use zinc lozenges are also more likely to have distorted taste and irritation in their mouths. The zinc might work for your cold, but it could make you prone to puking and not able to taste as well. Hmmm.

In fact, zinc's terrible taste actually hurts the science in these studies. Since the placebo pill did not taste like a gym sock, the study participants who got the zinc probably knew what they were taking. When people in a study know whether or not they are getting the thing being studied, the results are not as trustworthy.

There is an added zinc-related caution. In studies of zinc nasal gel, the gel improves cold symptoms and shortens colds, but it can permanently damage your sense of smell. Losing your sense of smell (and your sense of taste, which is affected by how well you can smell) is not a good price to pay for shortening your cold! Makers of a zinc nasal gel have actually paid out over $12 million in lawsuits to people with damaged senses of smell.

The bottom line is that zinc might help your cold, but it could also make you feel nauseous and alter your sense of taste. You might think zinc is worth a try, but you should know that zinc's benefits might not come so easily.

Acknowledgments

Both of us would like to say thank you to Jacob Brenner, who spent a summer helping us do much of the research behind this book. Additionally, we would like to thank the Indiana University School of Medicine Department of Pediatrics and the Division of Children's Health Services Research, as well as Riley Hospital for Children for their support. We are so appreciative of our agents, Sheree Bykofsky and Janet Rosen, as well as our editor, Alyse Diamond, who is also our go-to person for lunch when we are lucky enough to head to New York City.

Aaron would additionally like to thank his family and friends for their unending love and support. He is especially grateful for Jacob, who makes him think, Noah, who makes him laugh, and Sydney, who always holds his hand. He still marvels that he is married to Aimee, whom he loves madly, and who tolerates him better than anyone else in the world.

Rachel thanks Joe Fick, who takes good care of all living things in his sphere, including her. She also gives thanks to her wonderful family. Tom and Jacki Vreeman are not responsible for her desire to debunk parental wisdom except in that they raised a well-educated, independent thinker, and for this Rachel thanks them especially. Rachel appreciates her cheering section on both sides of the ocean, with special thanks to her favorite women (especially Elizabeth, Maria, Jessica, Lorrie, and Jessica), the Vreeman tribe, the Fountain Square Supper Club, and the I.U. Kenya team. Rachel also acknowledges that Aaron is almost always right.

References

You know what'll really get rid of that cold? . . . Acupuncture!

Kawakita, K., T. Shichidou, E. Inoue, T. Nabeta, H. Kitakouji, S. Aizawa, A. Nishida, N. Yamaguchi, N. Takahashi, T. Yano, and S. Tanzawa. "Preventive and Curative Effects of Acupuncture on the Common Cold: A Multicentre Randomized Controlled Trial in Japan." *Complement Ther Med* 12, no. 4 (2004): 181–8.

Seki, K. "Examination of Effect of Acupuncture Treatment to Cold." *Oriental Med* 20 (1992): 71–3.

Tan, D. "Treatment of Fever Due to Exopathic Wind-Cold by Rapid Acupuncture." *J Tradit Chin Med* 12, no. 4 (1992): 267–71.

Tokuchi, J., and S. Tanzawa. "Remarkable Improvement of Chronic Cold Syndrome by the Application of Acupuncture Therapy to a Patient with 'Fei Qi Ying Liang Xiu Zhen.' " *J Jpn Soci Acupunct and Moxibustion* 50 (2000): 463–9.

ADHD medication will stunt your child's growth

Faraone, S. V., and E. E. Giefer. "Long-Term Effects of Methylphenidate Transdermal Delivery System Treatment of ADHD on Growth." *J Am Acad Child Psy* 46, no 9 (2007): 1138–47.

Faraone, S. V., and J. Biederman et al. "Effect of Stimulants on Height and Weight: A Review of the Literature." *J Am Acad Child Psy* 47, no. 9 (2008): 994–1009.

Matlen, T. "Do Stimulants Stunt Growth?—ADHD." HealthCentral.com (2010), http://www.healthcentral.com/adhd/c/57718/28350/stimulants-growth

Poulton, A. "Growth on Stimulant Medication; Clarifying the Confusion: A Review." Archives of Disease in Childhood 90, no. 8 (2005): 801–6.

Poulton, A.S., and R. Nanan. "Prior Treatment with Stimulant Medication: A Much Neglected Confounder of Studies of Growth in Children with Attention-Deficit/Hyperactivity Disorder." *J Child Adolec Psychopharmacol* 18, no. 4 (2008): 385–7.

Spencer, T. J., and J. Biederman et al. "Growth Deficits in ADHD Children Revisited: Evidence for Disorder-Associated Growth Delays?" *J Am Acad Child Psy* 35, no. 11 (1996): 1460–9.

The air you breathe will make you sick . . .
if you're near a sniffler and sneezer

Caruso, T. J., and J. M. Gwaltney, Jr. "Treatment of the Common Cold with Echinacea: A Structured Review." *Clin Infect Dis* 40, no. 6 (2005): 807–10.

Dick, E. C., L. C. Jennings, K. A. Mink, C. D. Wartgow, and S. L. Inhorn. "Aerosol Transmission of Rhinovirus Colds." *J Infect Dis* 156, no. 3 (1987): 442–8.

Escombe, A. R., C. C. Oeser, R. H. Gilman, M. Navincopa, E. Ticona, W. Pan, C. Martinez, J. Chacaltana, R. Rodriguez, D. A. Moore, J. S. Friedland, and C. A. Evans. "Natural Ventilation for the Prevention of Airborne Contagion." *PLoS Med* 4, no. 2 (2007): e68.

Gwaltney, J. M., and J. O. Hendley. "Rhinovirus Transmission: One if by Air, Two if by Hand." *Trans Am Clin Climatol Assoc* 89 (1978): 194–200.

Gwaltney, J. M., Jr., P. B. Moskalski, and J. O. Hendley. "Hand-to-Hand Transmission of Rhinovirus Colds." *Ann Intern Med* 88, no. 4 (1978): 463–7.

Hendley, J. O., R. P. Wenzel, and J. M. Gwaltney, Jr. "Transmission of Rhinovirus Colds by Self-Inoculation." *N Engl J Med* 288, no. 26 (1973): 1361–4.

Myatt, T. A., S. L. Johnston, Z. Zuo, M. Wand, T. Kebadze, S. Rudnick, and D. K. Milton. "Detection of Airborne Rhinovirus and Its Relation to Outdoor Air Supply in Office Environments." *Am J Respir Crit Care Med* 169, no. 11 (2004): 1187–90.

Nardell, E. A., J. Keegan, S. A. Cheney, and S. C. Etkind. "Airborne Infection. Theoretical Limits of Protection Achievable by Building Ventilation." *Am Rev Respir Dis* 144, no. 2 (1991): 302–6.

Nielsen, P. V. "Control of Airborne Infectious Diseases in Ventilated Spaces." *J R Soc Interface* 6 Suppl 6 (2009): S747–55.

Noakes, C. J., C. B. Beggs, P. A. Sleigh, and K. G. Kerr. "Modelling the Transmission of Airborne Infections in Enclosed Spaces." *Epidemiol Infect* 134, no. 5 (2006): 1082–91.

Samet, J. M. "How Do We Catch Colds?" *Am J Respir Crit Care Med* 169, no. 11 (2004): 1175–6.

I have just the thing for that cold . . . Airborne

"Airborne Effects Unstudied." *Los Angeles Times* (2008), http://www.latimes.com/features/printedition/health/la-he-airborne18feb18,1,5237479.story.

Barrett, K. "Airborne to Refund Consumers." ABC News Health (2008), http://abcnews.go.com/Health/ColdFlu/story?id=4380374&page=1.

Center for Science in the Public Interest. "Airborne Agrees to Pay $23.3 Million to Settle Lawsuit over False Advertising of Its 'Miracle Cold Buster.'" 2008, http://www.cspinet.org/new/200803032.html.

Crislip, M. "Deconstructing Airborne: How to Recognize Medical Nonsense." Pediatrics for Parents, http://www.pedsforparents.com/articles/3293.shtml. (Accessed 6/2/2010.)

"Does Airborne Really Stave Off Colds?" ABCNews.com (2006), http://abcnews.go.com/GMA/OnCall/story?id=1664514&page=1.

"Makers of Airborne Settle FTC Charges of Deceptive Advertising." Federal Trade Commission, 2008.

Nizza, M. "Makers of Airborne Settle False-Ad Suit with Refunds." *New York Times* (2008), http://thelede.blogs.nytimes.com/2008/03/04makers-of-airborne-settle-false-ad-suit-with-refunds/?ex=1205298000&en=10959dcfad803f0e&ei=5070&emc=etal.

Spiesel, S. "Your Health This Week." *Slate*, 14 March 2008.

Taylor, E. N., M. J. Stampfer, and G. C. Curhan. "Dietary Factors and the Risk of Incident Kidney Stones in Men: New Insights after 14 Years of Follow-Up." *J Am Soc Nephrol* 15, no. 12 (2004): 3225–32.

Airplane travel will make you sick

Baker, M. G., C. N. Thornley, C. Mills, S. Roberts, S. Perera, J. Peters, A. Kelso, I. Barr, and N. Wilson. "Transmission of Pandemic a/H1n1 2009 Influenza on Passenger Aircraft: Retrospective Cohort Study." *BMJ* 340 (2010): c2424.

DeHart, R. L. "Health Issues of Air Travel." *Annu Rev Public Health* 24 (2003): 133–51.

Forman, J. "Woman Claims Airplane Ride Disabled Her." *NWCN.com* (2010), http://www.nwcn.com/home/Woman-claims-airplane-ride-disabled-her-83862407.html.

Holmes, J. D., and G. C. Simmons. "Gastrointestinal Illness Associated with a Long-Haul Flight." *Epidemiol Infect* 137, no. 3 (2009): 441–7.

Leder, K., and D. Newman. "Respiratory Infections During Air Travel." *Intern Med J* 35, no. 1 (2005): 50–5.

Samet, J. M. "How Do We Catch Colds?" *Am J Respir Crit Care Med* 169, no. 11 (2004): 1175–6.

Sohail, M. R., and P. R. Fischer. "Health Risks to Air Travelers." *Infect Dis Clin North Am* 19, no. 1 (2005): 67–84.

Wagner, B. G., B. J. Coburn, and S. Blower. "Calculating the Potential for Within-Flight Transmission of Influenza a (H1n1)." *BMC Med* 7 (2009): 81.

Weiner, R. "Biden: I Told Family to Avoid Planes, Subway over Swine Flu." *Huffington Post*, http://www.huffingtonpost.com/2009/04/30/biden-swine-flu-made-me-t_n_193473.html. (Accessed on 7/21/10.)

Aloe vera will heal a burn—TRUE

Gallagher, J., and M. Gray. "Is Aloe Vera Effective for Healing Chronic Wounds?" *J Wound Ostomy Continence Nurs* 30, no. 2 (2003): 68–71.

Hosseinimehr, S. J., G. Khorasani, M. Azadbakht, P. Zamani, M. Ghasemi, and A. Ahmadi. "Effect of Aloe Cream Versus Silver Sulfadiazine for Healing Burn Wounds in Rats." *Acta Dermatovenerol Croat* 18, no. 1 (2010): 2–7.

Khorasani, G., S. J. Hosseinimehr, M. Azadbakht, A. Zamani, and M. R. Mahdavi. "Aloe Versus Silver Sulfadiazine Creams for Second-Degree Burns: A Randomized Controlled Study." *Surg Today* 39, no. 7 (2009): 587–91.

Maenthaisong, R., N. Chaiyakunapruk, S. Niruntraporn, and C. Kongkaew. "The Efficacy of Aloe Vera Used for Burn Wound Healing: A Systematic Review." *Burns* 33, no. 6 (2007): 713–8.

Takzare, N., M. J. Hosseini, G. Hasanzadeh, H. Mortazavi, A. Takzare, and P. Habibi. "Influence of Aloe Vera Gel on Dermal Wound Healing Process in Rat." *Toxicol Mech Methods* 19, no. 1 (2009): 73–7.

Visuthikosol, V., B. Chowchuen, Y. Sukwanarat, S. Sriurairatana, and V. Boonpucknavig. "Effect of Aloe Vera Gel to Healing of Burn Wound a Clinical and Histologic Study." *J Med Assoc Thai* 78, no. 8 (1995): 403–9.

Antibiotics kill the germs that cause colds and the flu

"Get Smart: Know When Antibiotics Work." Centers for Disease Control and Prevention, http://www.cdc.gov/features/getsmart/. (Accessed 6/11/10.)

Greene, A. "Antibiotics and the Common Cold." DrGreene.com, http://www .drgreene.com/qa/antibiotics-and-common-cold. (Accessed 6/11/10.)

"Information from Your Family Doctor. Antibiotics: When They Can and Can't Help." *Am Fam Physician* 74, no. 7 (2006): 1188.

Once an individual has started a course of antibiotics, he is no longer contagious

Call, S. A., M. A. Vollenweider, C. A. Hornung, D. L. Simel, and W. P. Mc-Kinney. "Does This Patient Have Influenza?" *JAMA* 293, no. 8 (2005): 987–97.

De Serres, G., I. Rouleau, M. E. Hamelin, C. Quach, D. Skowronski, L. Flamand, N. Boulianne, Y. Li, J. Carbonneau, A. Bourgault, M. Couillard, H. Charest, and G. Boivin. "Contagious Period for Pandemic (H1n1) 2009." *Emerg Infect Dis* 16, no. 5 (2010): 783–8.

Kimura, R., H. Migita, K. Kadonosono, and E. Uchio. "Is It Possible to Detect the Presence of Adenovirus in Conjunctiva Before the Onset of Conjunctivitis?" *Acta Ophthalmol* 87, no. 1 (2009): 44–7.

Lau, L. L., B. J. Cowling, V. J. Fang, K. H. Chan, E. H. Lau, M. Lipsitch, C. K. Cheng, P. M. Houck, T. M. Uyeki, J. S. Peiris, and G. M. Leung. "Viral Shedding and Clinical Illness in Naturally Acquired Influenza Virus Infections." *J Infect Dis* 201, no. 10 (2010): 1509–16.

Musher, D. M. "How Contagious Are Common Respiratory Tract Infections?" *N Engl J Med* 348, no. 13 (2003): 1256–66.

Schmitt, B. D. "Your Child's Health." Bantam Books, http://www.cpnonline .org/CRS/CRS/pa_incubate_hhg.htm. (Accessed 6/7/10.)

An apple a day keeps the doctor away

Aprikian, O., M. Levrat-Verny, C. Besson, J. Busserolles, C. Remesy, and C. Demigne. "Apple Favourably Affects Parameters of Cholesterol Metabolism and of Anti-Oxidative Protection in Cholesterol Fed Rats." *Food Chem* 75 (2001): 445–52.

Aprikian, O., J. Busserolles, C. Manach, A. Mazur, C. Morand, M. J. Davicco, C. Besson, Y. Rayssiguier, C. Remesy, and C. Demigne. "Lyophilized Apple Counteracts the Development of Hypercholesterolemia, Oxidative Stress, and Renal Dysfunction in Obese Zucker Rats." *J Nutr* 132, no. 7 (2002): 1969–76.

Boyer, J., and R. H. Liu. "Apple Phytochemicals and Their Health Benefits." *Nutr J* 3 (2004): 5.

DuPont, M. S., R. N. Bennett, F. A. Mellon, and G. Williamson. "Polyphenols from Alcoholic Apple Cider Are Absorbed, Metabolized and Excreted by Humans." *J Nutr* 132, no. 2 (2002): 172–5.

Eberhardt, M. V., C. Y. Lee, and R. H. Liu. "Antioxidant Activity of Fresh Apples." *Nature* 405, no. 6789 (2000): 903–4.

Feskanich, D., R. G. Ziegler, D. S. Michaud, E. L. Giovannucci, F. E. Speizer, W. C. Willett, and G. A. Colditz. "Prospective Study of Fruit and Vegetable Consumption and Risk of Lung Cancer Among Men and Women." *J Natl Cancer Inst* 92, no. 22 (2000): 1812–23.

Hollman, P. C., J. M. van Trijp, M. N. Buysman, M. S. van der Gaag, M. J. Mengelers, J. H. de Vries, and M. B. Katan. "Relative Bioavailability of the Antioxidant Flavonoid Quercetin from Various Foods in Man." *FEBS Lett* 418, no. 1–2 (1997): 152–6.

Jedrychowski, W., U. Maugeri, T. Popiela, J. Kulig, E. Sochacka-Tatara, A. Pac, A. Sowa, and A. Musial. "Case-Control Study on Beneficial Effect of Regular Consumption of Apples on Colorectal Cancer Risk in a Population with Relatively Low Intake of Fruits and Vegetables." *Eur J Cancer Prev* 19, no. 1 (2010): 42–7.

Knekt, P., R. Jarvinen, A. Reunanen, and J. Maatela. "Flavonoid Intake and Coronary Mortality in Finland: A Cohort Study." *BMJ* 312, no. 7029 (1996): 478–81.

Knekt, P., R. Jarvinen, R. Seppanen, M. Hellovaara, L. Teppo, E. Pukkala, and A. Aromaa. "Dietary Flavonoids and the Risk of Lung Cancer and Other Malignant Neoplasms." *Am J Epidemiol* 146, no. 3 (1997): 223–30.

Knekt, P., J. Kumpulainen, R. Jarvinen, H. Rissanen, M. Heliovaara, A. Reunanen, T. Hakulinen, and A. Aromaa. "Flavonoid Intake and Risk of Chronic Diseases." *Am J Clin Nutr* 76, no. 3 (2002): 560–8.

Le Marchand, L., S. P. Murphy, J. H. Hankin, L. R. Wilkens, and L. N. Kolonel. "Intake of Flavonoids and Lung Cancer." *J Natl Cancer Inst* 92, no. 2 (2000): 154–60.

Leontowicz, H., S. Gorinstein, A. Lojek, M. Leontowicz, Ci, M. z, R. Soliva-Fortuny, Y. S. Park, S. T. Jung, S. Trakhtenberg, and O. Martin-Belloso. "Comparative Content of Some Bioactive Compounds in Apples, Peaches and Pears and Their Influence on Lipids and Antioxidant Capacity in Rats." *J Nutr Biochem* 13, no. 10 (2002): 603–10.

Liu, R. H., M. Eberhardt, and C. Lee. "Antioxidant and Antiproliferative Activities of Selected New York Apple Cultivars." *New York Fruit Quarterly* 9 (2001): 15–17.

Sesso, H. D., J. M. Gaziano, S. Liu, and J. E. Buring. "Flavonoid Intake and the Risk of Cardiovascular Disease in Women." *Am J Clin Nutr* 77, no. 6 (2003): 1400–8.

Shmerling, R. H. "Putting the Apple-a-Day Adage to the Test." MSN Health and Fitness (2009), http://health.msn.com/nutrition/articlepage.aspx?cp-documentid =100211721.

Soler, C., J. M. Soriano, and J. Manes. "Apple-Products Phytochemicals and Processing: A Review." *Nat Prod Commun* 4, no. 5 (2009): 659–70.

Tabak, C., I. C. Arts, H. A. Smit, D. Heederik, and D. Kromhout. "Chronic Obstructive Pulmonary Disease and Intake of Catechins, Flavonols, and Flavones: The Morgen Study." *Am J Respir Crit Care Med* 164, no. 1 (2001): 61–4.

Wolfe, K., X. Wu, and R. H. Liu. "Antioxidant Activity of Apple Peels." *J Agric Food Chem* 51, no. 3 (2003): 609–14.

Woods, R. K., E. H. Walters, J. M. Raven, R. Wolfe, P. D. Ireland, F. C. Thien, and M. J. Abramson. "Food and Nutrient Intakes and Asthma Risk in Young Adults." *Am J Clin Nutr* 78, no. 3 (2003): 414–21.

Artificial sweeteners will give you cancer

Associated Press. "Artificial Sweetener Cleared of Cancer Link." MSNBC Health (2006), http://www.msnbc.msn.com/id/12155793/.

Center for Science in the Public Interest. "FDA Should Reconsider Aspartame Cancer Risk, Say Experts." (2007), http://www.cspinet.org/new/200706251.html.

Dean, C., and E. Meininger. "Will N.M. Be First State to Ban Aspartame?" NewsWithViews.com, http://www.newswithviews.com/Dean/carolyn26.htm. (Accessed 7/22/10.)

Gorman, C. "A Web of Deceit." *Time* (1999), http://www.time.com/time/magazine/article/0,9171,990167,00.html.

Halber, D. "Study Reaffirms Safety of Aspartame." *TechTalk* (1998). http://web.archive.org./web/20050207034647/http://web.mit.edu/newsoffice/tt/1998/sep16/aspartame.html.

Joe, D. B. "5 Things They Say Give You Cancer (and Why They're Wrong)." Cracked.com, http://www.cracked.com/article_17578_5-things-they-say-give-you-cancer-why-theyre-wrong.html.

Lim, U., A. F. Subar, T. Mouw, P. Hartge, L. M. Morton, R. Stolzenberg-Solomon, D. Campbell, A. R. Hollenbeck, and A. Schatzkin. "Consumption of Aspartame-Containing Beverages and Incidence of Hematopoietic and Brain Malignancies." *Cancer Epidemiol Biomarkers Prev* 15, no. 9 (2006): 1654–9.

Miller, E. "Aspartame: Fact or Fiction?" In *Emma Miller*, 2010. http://emmacmiller.blogspot.com/2010/06/aspartame-fact-or-fiction.html.

National Cancer Institute. "Artificial Sweeteners and Cancer." http://www.cancer.gov/cancertopics/factsheet/Risk/artificial-sweeteners. (Accessed 6/19/10.)

Suddath, C. "Are Artificial Sweeteners Really That Bad for You?" *Time* (2009), http://www.time.com/time/health/article/0,8599,1931116,00.html. (Accessed 6/19/10.)

Weihrauch, M. R., and V. Diehl. "Artificial Sweeteners—Do They Bear a Carcinogenic Risk?" *Ann Oncol* 15, no. 10 (2004): 1460–5.

The door handle is the dirtiest fixture in the bathroom

"The Germiest Places in America." Health.com, http://living.health.com/2008/03/12/the-germiest-places-in-america/. (Accessed 7/1/10.)

"Germs, Hands and Your Health." Handlerusa.com, http://www.handlerusa.com/germsandhealth.php. (Accessed 8/4/10.)

The Informed Patient. "Where the Worst Germs Lurk." *Wall Street Journal* (2009), http://online.wsj.com/article/SB10001424052748703787204574440983321928144.html.

Palenik, C. J. "Dr. Germ: Charles P. Gerba." *Dental Office Magazine*, 28 December 2007.

Reynolds, K. A., P. M. Watt, S. A. Boone, and C. P. Gerba. "Occurrence of Bacteria and Biochemical Markers on Public Surfaces." *Int J Environ Health Res* 15, no. 3 (2005): 225–34.

Roufos, A. "Germ and Bacteria Hot-Spots: 12 Things You Should Know." *Fitness*, http://features.fitnessmagazine.com/12ThingsYouShouldKnowAboutGermandBacteriaHotSpots.html. (Accessed 6/30/10.)

Air dryers will keep your hands cleaner than paper towels

Gustafson, D. R., E. A. Vetter, D. R. Larson, D. M. Ilstrup, M. D. Maker, R. L. Thompson, and F. R. Cockerill, III. "Effects of 4 Hand-Drying Methods for Removing Bacteria from Washed Hands: A Randomized Trial." *Mayo Clin Proc* 75, no. 7 (2000): 705–8.

Harrison, W. A., C. J. Griffith, T. Ayers, and B. Michaels. "Bacterial Transfer and Cross-Contamination Potential Associated with Paper-Towel Dispensing." *Am J Infect Control* 31, no. 7 (2003): 387–91.

Harrison, W. A., C. J. Griffith, B. Michaels, and T. Ayers. "Technique to Determine Contamination Exposure Routes and the Economic Efficiency of Folded Paper-Towel Dispensing." *Am J Infect Control* 31, no. 2 (2003): 104–8.

Main, E. "This or That: Paper Towels vs. Electric Dryers." Rodale.com, http://www.rodale.com/electric-hand-dryers. (Accessed 7/1/10.)

Redway, K. "A Comparative Study of Three Different Hand Drying Methods: Paper Towel, Warm Air Dryer, Jet Air Dryer." University of Westminster, London, 2008.

TUV Produkt and Umwelt GmbH. "Concerning a Study Conducted with Regard to the Different Methods Used for Drying Hands." 2005.

Yamamoto, Y., K. Ugai, and Y. Takahashi. "Efficiency of Hand Drying for Removing Bacteria from Washed Hands: Comparison of Paper Towel Drying with Warm Air Drying." *Infect Control Hosp Epidemiol* 26, no. 3 (2005): 316–20.

The bubbles in soda will make your bones brittle

Heaney, R. P., and K. Rafferty. "Carbonated Beverages and Urinary Calcium Excretion." *Am J Clin Nutr* 74, no. 3 (2001): 343–7.

Mahmood, M., A. Saleh, F. Al-Alawi, and F. Ahmed. "Health Effects of Soda Drinking in Adolescent Girls in the United Arab Emirates." *J Crit Care* 23, no. 3 (2008): 434–40.

McGartland, C., P. J. Robson, L. Murray, G. Cran, M. J. Savage, D. Watkins, M. Rooney, and C. Boreham. "Carbonated Soft Drink Consumption and Bone Mineral Density in Adolescence: The Northern Ireland Young Hearts Project." *J Bone Miner Res* 18, no. 9 (2003): 1563–9.

Robb-Nicholson, C. "By the Way, Doctor. I've Heard That Club Soda, Seltzer Water, and Sparkling Mineral Waters Rob the Bones of Calcium? Is This True?" *Harv Womens Health Watch* 17, no. 5 (2010): 8.

Tucker, K. L., K. Morita, N. Qiao, M. T. Hannan, L. A. Cupples, and D. P. Kiel. "Colas, but Not Other Carbonated Beverages, Are Associated with Low Bone Mineral Density in Older Women: The Framingham Osteoporosis Study." *Am J Clin Nutr* 84, no. 4 (2006): 936–42.

Weil, A. "Confused About Carbonation?" DrWeil.com, http://www.drweil.com/drw/u/id/QAA157077. (Accessed 6/22/10.)

Caffeine stunts your growth

Bauer., J. "Fact or Fiction: Common Diet Myths Dispelled." http://today.msnbc.msn.com/id/16280050/. (Accessed 6/24/10.)

Heaney, R. P. "Effects of Caffeine on Bone and the Calcium Economy." *Food Chem Toxicol* 40, no. 9 (2002): 1263–70.

O'Connor, A. "The Claim: Drinking Coffee Can Stunt a Child's Growth." *New York Times* (2005), http://www.nytimes.com/2005/10/18/health/18real.html?_r=1.

Paul, D. C., and C. W. Goff. "Comparative Effects of Caffeine, Its Analogues and Calcium Deficiency on Cytokinesis." *Exp Cell Res* 78, no. 2 (1973): 399–413.

Cancer is unpreventable

"Antioxidants and Cancer Prevention: Fact Sheet." National Cancer Institute, http://www.cancer.gov/cancertopics/factsheet/prevention/antioxidants. (Accessed 6/16/10.)

Boyer, J., Liu. "Apple Phytochemicals and Their Health Benefits." *Nutr J* 3 (2004): 5.

"Cancer Prevention Overiew." National Cancer Institute, http://www.cancer.gov/cancertopics/pdq/prevention/overview/healthprofessional. (Accessed 6/16/10.)

Jedrychowski, W., U. Maugeri, T. Popiela, J. Kulig, E. Sochacka-Tatara, A. Pac, A. Sowa, and A. Musial. "Case-Control Study on Beneficial Effect of Regular Consumption of Apples on Colorectal Cancer Risk in a Population with Relatively Low Intake of Fruits and Vegetables." *Eur J Cancer Prev* 19, no. 1 (2010): 42–7.

Nelson, S. "How to Prevent Cancer." *Causecast* (2010), http://www.tonic.com/article/how-to-prevent-cancer/.

Soler, C., J. M. Soriano, and J. Manes. "Apple-Products Phytochemicals and Processing: A Review." *Nat Prod Commun* 4, no. 5 (2009): 659–70.

Celery has negative calories

"Celery and Negative Calories." Snopes.com. (2010), http://www.snopes.com/food/ingredient/celery.asp. (Accessed 10/6/10.)

"Does Chewing Celery Consume More Calories than It Provides." StraightDope.com. (2010), http://www.straightdope.com/columns/read/2507/does-chewing-celery-consume-more-calories-than-it-provides. (Accessed 10/6/10.)

"Is It True That Celery Has Negative Calories." Answers.com. (2010), http://wiki.answers.com/Q/Is_it_true_that_celery_has_negative_calories. (Accessed 10/6/10.)

"Myth or Fact: Celery Has Negative Calories." FitDay.com. (2010), http://www.fitday.com/fitness-articles/nutrition/healthy-eating/myth-or-fact-celery-has-negative-calories.html. (Accessed 10/6/10.)

Cell phones cause brain tumors

Ahlbom, A., M. Feychting, A. Green, L. Kheifets, D. A. Savitz, and A. J. Swerdlow. "Epidemiologic Evidence on Mobile Phones and Tumor Risk: A Review." *Epidemiology* 20, no. 5 (2009): 639–52.

Betts, K. S. "Electromagnetic Fields: Conference, Hearing Call Up Cell Phone Use." *Environ Health Perspect* 117, no. 11 (2009): A486.

Hardell, L., and M. Carlberg. "Mobile Phones, Cordless Phones and the Risk for Brain Tumours." *Int J Oncol* 35, no. 1 (2009): 5–17.

Hardell, L., M. Carlberg, and K. Hansson Mild. "Use of Cellular Telephones and Brain Tumour Risk in Urban and Rural Areas." *Occup Environ Med* 62, no. 6 (2005): 390–4.

Hepworth, S. J., M. J. Schoemaker, K. R. Muir, A. J. Swerdlow, M. J. van Tongeren, and P. A. McKinney. "Mobile Phone Use and Risk of Glioma in Adults: Case-Control Study." *BMJ* 332, no. 7546 (2006): 883–7.

Kundi, M. "The Controversy About a Possible Relationship Between Mobile Phone Use and Cancer." *Environ Health Perspect* 117, no. 3 (2009): 316–24.

Mead, M. N. "Strong Signal for Cell Phone Effects." *Environ Health Perspect* 116, no. 10 (2008): A422.

Myung, S. K., W. Ju, D. D. McDonnell, Y. J. Lee, G. Kazinets, C. T. Cheng, and J. M. Moskowitz. "Mobile Phone Use and Risk of Tumors: A Meta-Analysis." *J Clin Oncol* 27, no. 33 (2009): 5565–72.

Soller, K. "Kids, Put Down Your Cell Phones!" *Newsweek* 152, no. 7–8 (2008): 63.

Takebayashi, T., N. Varsier, Y. Kikuchi, K. Wake, M. Taki, S. Watanabe, S. Akiba, and N. Yamaguchi. "Mobile Phone Use, Exposure to Radiofrequency Electromagnetic Field, and Brain Tumour: A Case-Control Study." *Br J Cancer* 98, no. 3 (2008): 652–9.

Thun, M. J. "Jury Still Out on Cell Phone-Cancer Connection." *Cancer* 116, no. 9 (2010): 2067.

Cheese makes you constipated

Anthoni, S., E. Savilahti, H. Rautelin, and K. L. Kolho. "Milk Protein Igg and Iga: The Association with Milk-Induced Gastrointestinal Symptoms in Adults." *World J Gastroenterol* 15, no. 39 (2009): 4915–8.

"Constipation." National Digestive Diseases Information Clearinghouse (NDDIC), http://digestive.niddk.nih.gov/ddiseases/pubs/constipation/. (Accessed 6/18/10.)

Corkins, M. R. "Are Diet and Constipation Related in Children?" *Nutr Clin Pract* 20, no. 5 (2005): 536–9.

"Foods That Cause Constipation." Colon Cleansing & Constipation Resource Center, http://www.fairyshare.com/watch-d418daca26b74d750#.

Greene, A. "Milk and Constipation." DrGreene.com, http://www.fairyshare.com/watch-d418daca26b74d750#. (Accessed 6/19/10.)

Sandler, R. S., M. C. Jordan, and B. J. Shelton. "Demographic and Dietary Determinants of Constipation in the US Population." *Am J Public Health* 80, no. 2 (1990): 185–9.

I have just the thing for that cold . . . Chicken Soup—TRUE

Hopkins, A. B. "Chicken Soup Cure May Not Be a Myth." *Nurse Pract* 28, no. 6 (2003): 16.

Ohry, A., and J. Tsafrir. "Is Chicken Soup an Essential Drug?" *CMAJ* 161, no. 12 (1999): 1532–3.

Rennard, B. O., R. F. Ertl, G. L. Gossman, R. A. Robbins, and S. I. Rennard. "Chicken Soup Inhibits Neutrophil Chemotaxis in Vitro." *Chest* 118, no. 4 (2000): 1150–7.

Saketkhoo, K., A. Januszkiewicz, and M. A. Sackner. "Effects of Drinking Hot Water, Cold Water, and Chicken Soup on Nasal Mucus Velocity and Nasal Airflow Resistance." *Chest* 74, no. 4 (1978): 408–10.

Chocolate or fried foods cause acne

"Acne Myths." AcneNet, http://www.skincarephysicians.com/acnenet/myths .html. (Accessed 6/24/10.)

Davidovici, B. B., and R. Wolf. "The Role of Diet in Acne: Facts and Controversies." *Clin Dermatol* 28, no. 1 (2010): 12–6.

El-Akawi, Z., N. Abdel-Latif Nemr, K. Abdul-Razzak, and M. Al-Aboosi. "Factors Believed by Jordanian Acne Patients to Affect Their Acne Condition." *East Mediterr Health J* 12, no. 6 (2006): 840–6.

Ferdowsian, H. R., and S. Levin. "Does Diet Really Affect Acne?" *Skin Therapy Lett* 15, no. 3 (2010): 1–2, 5.

Magin, P., D. Pond, W. Smith, and A. Watson. "A Systematic Review of the Evidence for 'Myths and Misconceptions' in Acne Management: Diet, Face-Washing and Sunlight." *Fam Pract* 22, no. 1 (2005): 62–70.

Wolf, R., H. Matz, and E. Orion. "Acne and Diet." *Clin Dermatol* 22, no. 5 (2004): 387–93.

Cold weather (and being underdressed for cold weather) will make you sick

Brenner, I. K., J. W. Castellani, C. Gabaree, A. J. Young, J. Zamecnik, R. J. Shephard, and P. N. Shek. "Immune Changes in Humans During Cold Exposure: Effects of Prior Heating and Exercise." *J Appl Physiol* 87, no. 2 (1999): 699–710.

Douglas, R. G., Jr. "Pathogenesis of Rhinovirus Common Colds in Human Voluteers." *Ann Otol Rhinol Laryngol* 79, no. 3 (1970): 563–71.

Eccles, R. "An Explanation for the Seasonality of Acute Upper Respiratory Tract Viral Infections." *Acta Otolaryngol* 122, no. 2 (2002): 183–91.

Lee, G. M., J. F. Friedman, D. Ross-Degnan, P. L. Hibberd, and D. A. Goldmann. "Misconceptions About Colds and Predictors of Health Service Utilization." *Pediatrics* 111, no. 2 (2003): 231–6.

Lowen, A. C., S. Mubareka, J. Steel, and P. Palese. "Influenza Virus Transmission Is Dependent on Relative Humidity and Temperature." *PLoS Pathog* 3, no. 10 (2007): 1470–6.

Melone, L. "Can the Cold Give You a Cold?" EverydayHealth.com, http://www.everydayhealth.com/cold-and-flu/colds-and-the-weather.aspx. (Accessed 6/1/10.)

Mirkin, G. "Catch a Cold." http://www.drmirkin.com/morehealth/9941.html.

O'Connor, A. "The Claim: You Lose Most of Your Body Heat through Your Head." *New York Times*, 28 October 2004.

Pretorius, T., G. K. Bristow, A. M. Steinman, and G. G. Giesbrecht. "Thermal Effects of Whole Head Submersion in Cold Water on Nonshivering Humans." *J Appl Physiol* 101, no. 2 (2006): 669–75.

Proud, D. "Upper Airway Viral Infections." *Pulm Pharmacol Ther* 21, no. 3 (2008): 468–73.

"U.S. Army Survival Manual: FM 21–76." In *U.S. Department of the Army*, ed. U.S. Department of the Army, 148, 1970.

Wimer, G. S. "Wearing a Cap, Thermoregulation, and Thermal Sensation During Running in a Hot Environment." *J Sports Med Phys Fitness* 49, no. 3 (2009): 272–7.

Zuger, A. "You'll Catch Your Death!' An Old Wives' Tale? Well . . ." NYTimes.com (2010), http://www.nytimes.com/2003/03/04/science/you-ll-catch-your-death-an-old-wives-tale-well.html. (Accessed 10/7/10.)

I have just the thing for that cold . . . Over-the-Counter Cough and Cold Medicines

Arroll, B. "Non-Antibiotic Treatments for Upper-Respiratory Tract Infections (Common Cold)." *Respir Med* 99, no. 12 (2005): 1477–84.

Bell, E. A., and D. E. Tunkel. "Over-the-Counter Cough and Cold Medications in Children: Are They Helpful?" *Otolaryngol Head Neck Surg* 142, no. 5 (2010): 647–50.

Bhatt-Mehta, V. "Over-the-Counter Cough and Cold Medicines: Should Parents Be Using Them for Their Children?" *Ann Pharmacother* 38, no. 11 (2004): 1964–6.

Chang, A. B., L. I. Landau, P. P. Van Asperen, N. J. Glasgow, C. F. Robertson, J. M. Marchant, and C. M. Mellis. "Cough in Children: Definitions and Clinical Evaluation." *Med J Aust* 184, no. 8 (2006): 398–403.

Chang, A. B., J. Peake, and M. S. McElrea. "Anti-Histamines for Prolonged Non-Specific Cough in Children." *Cochrane Database Syst Rev* 2 (2008): CD005604.

"FDA Statement Following CHPA's Announcement on Nonprescription Over-the-Counter Cough and Cold Medicines in Children." U.S. Food and Drug Administration (FDA), 2008.

"Infant Deaths Associated with Cough and Cold Medications—Two States, 2005." *MMWR Morb Mortal Wkly Rep* 56, no. 1 (2007): 1–4.

Johnson, G., and C. Helman. "Remedy or Cure? Lay Beliefs About Over-the-Counter Medicines for Coughs and Colds." *Br J Gen Pract* 54, no. 499 (2004): 98–102.

"Nonprescription Cough and Cold Medicine Use in Children." U.S. Food and Drug Administration (FDA), 2007.

Sharfstein, J. M., M. North, and J. R. Serwint. "Over the Counter but No Longer Under the Radar—Pediatric Cough and Cold Medications." *N Engl J Med* 357, no. 23 (2007): 2321–4.

Simasek, M., and D. A. Blandino. "Treatment of the Common Cold." *Am Fam Physician* 75, no. 4 (2007): 515–20.

Smith, S. M., K. Schroeder, and T. Fahey. "Over-the-Counter Medications for Acute Cough in Children and Adults in Ambulatory Settings." *Cochrane Database Syst Rev* 1 (2008): CD001831.

"Use of Codeine- and Dextromethorphan-Containing Cough Remedies in Children." American Academy of Pediatrics. Committee on Drugs. *Pediatrics* 99, no. 6 (1997): 918–20.

Cool mist will help your child's croup

Bourchier, D., K. P. Dawson, and D. M. Fergusson. "Humidification in Viral Croup: A Controlled Trial." *Aust Paediatr J* 20, no. 4 (1984): 289–91.

Henry, R. "Moist Air in the Treatment of Laryngotracheitis." *Arch Dis Child* 58, no. 8 (1983): 577.

Lenney, W., and A. D. Milner. "Treatment of Acute Viral Croup." *Arch Dis Child* 53, no. 9 (1978): 704–6.

Moore, M., and P. Little. "Humidified Air Inhalation for Treating Croup: A Systematic Review and Meta-Analysis." *Family Practice* 24, no. 4 (2007): 295–301.

Neto, G. M., O. Kentab, T. P. Klassen, and M. H. Osmond. "A Randomized Controlled Trial of Mist in the Acute Treatment of Moderate Croup." *Acad Emerg-Med* 9, no. 9 (2002): 873–79.

Scolnik, D., A. L. Coates, D. Stephens, Z. Da Silva, E. Lavine, and S. Schuh. "Controlled Delivery of High vs Low Humidity vs Mist Therapy for Croup in Emergency Departments: A Randomized Controlled Trial." *JAMA* 295, no. 11 (2006): 1274–80.

Skolnik, Neil S. "Treatment of Croup: A Critical Review." *Am J Dis Child* 143, no. 9 (1989): 1045–49.

Wolfsdorf, J., and D. L. Swift. "An Animal Model Simulating Acute Infective Upper Airway Obstruction of Childhood and Its Use in the Investigation of Croup Therapy." *Pediatr Res* 12, no. 11 (1978): 1062–5.

If you are sick, you should stay away from dairy products (milk makes you phelgmy)

Arney, W. K., and C. B. Pinnock. "The Milk Mucus Belief: Sensations Associated with the Belief and Characteristics of Believers." *Appetite* 20, no. 1 (1993): 53–60.

Bartley, J., and S. R. McGlashan. "Does Milk Increase Mucus Production?" *Med Hypotheses* 74, no. 4 (2010): 732–4.

Haas, F., M. C. Bishop, J. Salazar-Schicchi, K. V. Axen, D. Lieberman, and K. Axen. "Effect of Milk Ingestion on Pulmonary Function in Healthy and Asthmatic Subjects." *J Asthma* 28, no. 5 (1991): 349–55.

Lee, C., and A. J. Dozor. "Do You Believe Milk Makes Mucus?" *Arch Pediatr Adolesc Med* 158, no. 6 (2004): 601–3.

Nguyen, M. T. "Effect of Cow Milk on Pulmonary Function in Atopic Asthmatic Patients." *Ann Allergy Asthma Immunol* 79, no. 1 (1997): 62–4.

O'Connor, A. "The Claim: Milk Makes You Phlegmy." *New York Times*, 12 April 2010.

Pinnock, C. B., and W. K. Arney. "The Milk-Mucus Belief: Sensory Analysis Comparing Cow's Milk and a Soy Placebo." *Appetite* 20, no. 1 (1993): 61–70.

Pinnock, C. B., N. M. Graham, A. Mylvaganam, and R. M. Douglas. "Relationship Between Milk Intake and Mucus Production in Adult Volunteers Challenged with Rhinovirus-2." *Am Rev Respir Dis* 141, no. 2 (1990): 352–6.

Spock, B. *Spock's Baby and Child Care.* New York: Pocket Books, 1998.

Woods, R. K., J. M. Weiner, M. Abramson, F. Thien, and E. H. Walters. "Do Dairy Products Induce Bronchoconstriction in Adults with Asthma?" *J Allergy Clin Immunol* 101, no. 1 Pt 1 (1998): 45–50.

Wuthrich, B., A. Schmid, B. Walther, and R. Sieber. "Milk Consumption Does Not Lead to Mucus Production or Occurrence of Asthma." *J Am Coll Nutr* 24, no. 6 Suppl (2005): 547S–55S.

Kids in day care catch more colds

Collet, J. P., P. Burtin, and D. Floret. "Infectious Risk in Day-Nursery Children." *Rev Prat* 42, no. 14 (1992): 1797–803.

Dales, R. E., S. Cakmak, K. Brand, and S. Judek. "Respiratory Illness in Children Attending Daycare." *Pediatr Pulmonol* 38, no. 1 (2004): 64–9.

"Daycare Tots Under Age Two Most Apt to Catch Colds." Reuters Health, http://family.go.com/parenting/article-mm-77871-daycare-tots-under-age-two-most-apt-to-catch-colds-t/. (Accessed 6/9/10.)

"Is It True That Kids in Daycare Get Sick More Often than Kids Who Stay Home?" BabyCenter, http://www.babycenter.com/404_is-it-true-that-kids-in-day care-get-sick-more-often-than-kid_10323706.bc. (Accessed 6/9/10.)

Kamper-Jorgensen, M., L. G. Andersen, J. Simonsen, and S. Sorup. "Child Care Is Not a Substantial Risk Factor for Gastrointestinal Infection Hospitalization." *Pediatrics* 122, no. 6 (2008): e1168–73.

Kamper-Jorgensen, M., C. S. Benn, J. Simonsen, N. Thrane, and J. Wohlfahrt. "Clustering of Acute Respiratory Infection Hospitalizations in Childcare Facilities." *Acta Paediatr* 99, no. 6 (2010): 877–82.

Kamper-Jorgensen, M., J. Wohlfahrt, J. Simonsen, M. Gronbaek, and C. S. Benn. "Population-Based Study of the Impact of Childcare Attendance on Hospitalizations for Acute Respiratory Infections." *Pediatrics* 118, no. 4 (2006): 1439–46.

Deodorants and antiperspirants cause breast cancer

American Cancer Society. "Antiperspirants and Breast Cancer Risk." http://www.cancer.org/docroot/med/content/med_6_1x_antiperspirants.asp. (Accessed 6/19/10.)

Darbre, P. D. "Aluminium, Antiperspirants and Breast Cancer." *J Inorg Biochem* 99, no. 9 (2005): 1912–9.

———. "Underarm Cosmetics Are a Cause of Breast Cancer." *Eur J Cancer Prev* 10, no. 5 (2001): 389–93.

Gikas, P. D., L. Mansfield, and K. Mokbel. "Do Underarm Cosmetics Cause Breast Cancer?" *Int J Fertil Womens Med* 49, no. 5 (2004): 212–4.

McGrath, K. G. "An Earlier Age of Breast Cancer Diagnosis Related to More

Frequent Use of Antiperspirants/Deodorants and Underarm Shaving." *Eur J Cancer Prev* 12, no. 6 (2003): 479–85.

Surendran, A. "Studies Linking Breast Cancer to Deodorants Smell Rotten, Experts Say." *Nat Med* 10, no. 3 (2004): 216.

I have just the thing for that cold . . . Echinacea

Caruso, T. J., and J. M. Gwaltney, Jr. "Treatment of the Common Cold with Echinacea: A Structured Review." *Clin Infect Dis* 40, no. 6 (2005): 807–10.

Heaney, R. P. "Effects of Caffeine on Bone and the Calcium Economy." *Food Chem Toxicol* 40, no. 9 (2002): 1263–70.

Ross, S. M. "A Standardized Echinacea Extract Demonstrates Efficacy in the Prevention and Treatment of Colds in Athletes." *Holist Nurs Pract* 24, no. 2 (2010): 107–9.

Shah, S. A., S. Sander, C. M. White, M. Rinaldi, and C. I. Coleman. "Evaluation of Echinacea for the Prevention and Treatment of the Common Cold: A Meta-Analysis." *Lancet Infect Dis* 7, no. 7 (2007): 473–80.

Simasek, M., and D. A. Blandino. "Treatment of the Common Cold." *Am Fam Physician* 75, no. 4 (2007): 515–20.

Turner, R. B., R. Bauer, K. Woelkart, T. C. Hulsey, and J. D. Gangemi. "An Evaluation of Echinacea Angustifolia in Experimental Rhinovirus Infections." *N Engl J Med* 353, no. 4 (2005): 341–8.

von Maxen, A., and P. S. Schoenhoefer. "Benefit of Echinacea for the Prevention and Treatment of the Common Cold?" *Lancet Infect Dis* 8, no. 6 (2008): 346–7; author reply 47–8.

Woelkart, K., K. Linde, and R. Bauer. "Echinacea for Preventing and Treating the Common Cold." *Planta Med* 74, no. 6 (2008): 633–7.

Eggs give you high cholesterol

Behrenbeck, T. "Are Chicken Eggs Good or Bad for My Cholesterol?" MayoClinic .com, http://www.mayoclinic.com/health/cholesterol/hq00608. (Accessed 6/17/10.)

"Common Misconceptions About Cholesterol." American Heart Association, http://www.americanheart.org/presenter.jhtml?identifier=3006030.

Djousse, L., and J. M. Gaziano. "Egg Consumption and Risk of Heart Failure in the Physicians' Health Study." *Circulation* 117, no. 4 (2008): 512–6.

———. "Egg Consumption in Relation to Cardiovascular Disease and Mortality: The Physicians' Health Study." *Am J Clin Nutr* 87, no. 4 (2008): 964–9.

"Egg-Cellent News for Most, but Not Those with Diabetes. The Harmful Effects of Eggs Were Overblown, but the Studies Show That People with Diabetes Should Still Limit How Many They Eat." *Harv Health Lett* 33, no. 9 (2008): 6.

Fernandez, M. L. "Dietary Cholesterol Provided by Eggs and Plasma Lipoproteins in Healthy Populations." *Curr Opin Clin Nutr Metab Care* 9, no. 1 (2006): 8–12.

Hammett, A. "Shell out on Eggs." *The Sun* (London) (2009), http://www.thesun .co.uk/sol/homepage/woman/health/health/2273059/Eggs-dont-raise-cholestoral-levels-and-can-be-eaten-every-day-say-experts.html.

"I Have Heard That While Shrimp Is High in Fat and Cholesterol, It Is a Good

Kind of Fat That Is Healthy to Eat. Also, I Have Heard Conflicting Reports About Daily Consumption of Eggs—Some Say It's Not Recommended and Others Say It Won't Increase Serum Cholesterol Because the More Dietary Cholesterol One Consumes, the Less Cholesterol Is Produced by the Liver. Can You Explain?" *Heart Advis* 11, no. 10 (2008): 12.

Kritchevsky, S. B. "A Review of Scientific Research and Recommendations Regarding Eggs." *J Am Coll Nutr* 23, no. 6 Suppl (2004): 596S–600S.

McNamara, D. J. "Dietary Cholesterol and Blood Cholesterolemia: A Healthy Relationship." *World Rev Nutr Diet* 100 (2009): 55–62.

Mutungi, G., J. Ratliff, M. Puglisi, M. Torres-Gonzalez, U. Vaishnav, J. O. Leite, E. Quann, J. S. Volek, and M. L. Fernandez. "Dietary Cholesterol from Eggs Increases Plasma HDL Cholesterol in Overweight Men Consuming a Carbohydrate-Restricted Diet." *J Nutr* 138, no. 2 (2008): 272–6.

Parker-Pope. "8-Year-Olds on Statins? A New Plan Quickly Bites Back." In *Well: The New York Times Company*, 2008. http://www.nytimes.com/2008/07/08/health/08well.html?_r=2.

Sherrie. "Apparently, Consuming One Lousy Egg a Day Will Kill You . . ." In *Pinch of . . .* 2008. http://pinchof.blogspot.com/2008/04/apparently-consuming-one-lousy-egg-day.html.

"To Make an Omelet, You Have to Break Some Eggs. The Dangers of Eggs Aren't All They're Cracked Up to Be—Avoid Them If You Want, but It Isn't Necessary." *Harv Heart Lett* 16, no. 11 (2006): 3–4.

Raw eggs will give you salmonella

"Are Raw Eggs Safe to Eat? Ask the Fitness Nerd." Answerfitness.com. (2010), http://www.answerfitness.com/250/are-raw-eggs-safe-to-eat-fitness-nerd/. (Accessed 10/6/10.)

Claydon, J. "The Health Benefits of Raw Eggs." 2010, http://www.regenerative-nutrition.com/content.asp?id=268. (Accessed 10/6/10.)

Hope, B. K., A. R. Baker, E. D. Edel, A. T. Hogue, W. D. Schlosser, R. Whiting, R. M. McDowell, and R. A. Morales. "An Overview of the Salmonella Enteritidis Risk Assessment for Shell Eggs and Egg Products." *Risk Anal* 22, no. 2 (2002): 203–18.

"Myths and Facts About Eggs and Food Safety According to the American Egg Board/Egg Nutrition Center." Businesswire.com. (2010), http://findarticles.com/p/articles/mi_m0EIN/is_2001_June_14/ai_75535413/. (Accessed 10/6/10.)

If you stop exercising, your muscles will turn to fat

Austin, B. "Don't Let Your Body Go into Starvation Mode." *Wisconsin State Journal*, http://en.wikipedia.org/wiki/Physical_exercise#cite_ref-38.

"Turn Fat into Muscle? You've Heard the Phrase a Million Times, but Can You Really Turn Fat into Muscle?" *Muscle & Fitness*, http://findarticles.com/p/articles/mi_m0801/is_10_65/ai_n6237325/?tag=content.

Kruszelnicki, K. "Muscle Turns into Fat." ABC Science, http://www.abc.net.au/science/articles/2006/05/01/1613539.htm.

Don't cross your eyes . . . they'll get stuck that way!

Brain, M. "What if I Crossed My Eyes for 10 Minutes." Discovery Health (2010), http://health.howstuffworks.com/human-body/systems/eye/crossed-my-eyes.htm. (Accessed 10/7/10.)

"MYTH: If You Cross Your Eyes, They Can Stay like That." Globalnews.ca. (2010), http://www.globalnews.ca/money/story.html?id=2133165. (Accessed 10/7/10.)

Nelson, M. "You're Doing What?: Don't Cross Your Eyes or They Might Stay That Way." 2010, http://youredoingwhat.blogspot.com/2008/07/dont-cross-your-eyes-or-they-might-stay.html. (Accessed 10/7/10.)

Shmerling, R. "If You Cross Your Eyes Will They Get Stuck?" Health & Fitness—Health Topics (2010), http://health.msn.com/health-topics/articlepage.aspx?cp-documentid=100249849&pgnew=false. (Accessed 10/7/10.)

Tung, J. "The Truth About 12 Health Myths." RealSimple.com (2010), http://www.realsimple.com/health/first-aid-health-basics/old-wives-tales-retold-00000000040355/index.html. (Accessed 10/7/10.)

Rubbing your eyes is bad for you—TRUE

Greiner, J. V., D. G. Peace, R. S. Baird, and M. R. Allansmith. "Effects of Eye Rubbing on the Conjunctiva as a Model of Ocular Inflammation." *Am J Ophthalmol* 100, no. 1 (1985): 45–50.

Jacome, D. E. "Migraine Triggered by Rubbing the Eyes." *Headache* 38, no. 1 (1998): 50–2.

McMonnies, C. W. "Management of Chronic Habits of Abnormal Eye Rubbing." *Cont Lens Anterior Eye* 31, no. 2 (2008): 95–102.

Yeniad, B., N. Alparslan, and K. Akarcay. "Eye Rubbing as an Apparent Cause of Recurrent Keratoconus." *Cornea* 28, no. 4 (2009): 477–9.

Feed a cold, starve a fever

Bazar, K. A., A. J. Yun, and P. Y. Lee. " 'Starve a Fever and Feed a Cold': Feeding and Anorexia May Be Adaptive Behavioral Modulators of Autonomic and T Helper Balance." *Med Hypotheses* 64, no. 6 (2005): 1080–4.

Bishop, Eric. "Myth or Fact: Feed a Cold, Starve a Fever." DukeHealth.org (2008), http://www.dukehealth.org/health_library/health_articles/feed_a_cold.

van den Brink, G. R., D. E. van den Boogaardt, S. J. van Deventer, and M. P. Peppelenbosch. "Feed a Cold, Starve a Fever?" *Clin Diagn Lab Immunol* 9, no. 1 (2002): 182–3.

Yarnell, E. "Proposed Biomolecular Theory of Fasting During Fevers Due to Infection." *Altern Med Rev* 6, no. 5 (2001): 482–7.

If your temperature hits 104, you are going to have brain damage

Brody, J. "Personal Health." *New York Times* (1993), http://www.nytimes.com/1993/01/06/health/personal-health-798393.html?pagewanted=all.

Dinarello, C., and R. Porat. "Fever and Hyperthermia." In *Harrison's Principles of Internal Medicine*. http://www.accessmedicine.com/content.aspx?aID=2871336.

"Fever." NYTimes.com, http://health.nytimes.com/health/guides/symptoms/fever/overview.html. (Accessed 7/8/10.)

O'Connor, A. "The Claim: Rubbing Alcohol Can Help Cool a Fever." *New York Times* (2008), http://www.nytimes.com/2008/10/07/health/07real.html?adxnnl=1&adxnnlx=1278612157-i0mIxQVl8QWDl7VHoTXbHQ.

Sharma, H. S. "Heat-Related Deaths Are Largely Due to Brain Damage." *Indian J Med Res* 121, no. 5 (2005): 621–3.

Walsh, A., and H. Edwards. "Management of Childhood Fever by Parents: Literature Review." *J Adv Nurs* 54, no. 2 (2006): 217–27.

The flu is just a bad cold

"Cold Versus Flu." Centers for Disease Control and Prevention, http://www.cdc.gov/flu/about/qa/coldflu.htm. (Accessed 6/4/10.)

Eccles, R. "Understanding the Symptoms of the Common Cold and Influenza." *Lancet Infect Dis* 5, no. 11 (2005): 718–25.

Heikkinen, T., and A. Jarvinen. "The Common Cold." *Lancet* 361, no. 9351 (2003): 51–9.

I have just the thing for that cold . . . Garlic

Haake, P., T. H. Krueger, M. U. Goebel, K. M. Heberling, U. Hartmann, and M. Schedlowski. "Effects of Sexual Arousal on Lymphocyte Subset Circulation and Cytokine Production in Man." *Neuroimmunomodulation* 11, no. 5 (2004): 293–8.

Josling, P. "Preventing the Common Cold with a Garlic Supplement: A Double-Blind, Placebo-Controlled Survey." *Adv Ther* 18, no. 4 (2001): 189–93.

Lissiman, E., A. L. Bhasale, and M. Cohen. "Garlic for the Common Cold." *Cochrane Database Syst Rev* 3 (2009): CD006206.

If you have green snot, you need an antibiotic

"Antibiotics Slightly Effective for Purulent Rhinitis." *J Fam Pract* 55, no. 11 (2006): 944.

Arroll, B., and T. Kenealy. "Antibiotics for Acute Purulent Rhinitis." *BMJ* 325, no. 7376 (2002): 1311–2.

———. "Are Antibiotics Effective for Acute Purulent Rhinitis? Systematic Review and Meta-Analysis of Placebo Controlled Randomised Trials." *BMJ* 333, no. 7562 (2006): 279.

Arroll, B., T. Kenealy, and K. Falloon. "Are Antibiotics Indicated as an Initial Treatment for Patients with Acute Upper Respiratory Tract Infections? A Review." *N Z Med J* 121, no. 1284 (2008): 64–70.

Cates, C. J. "Antibiotics and Acute Purulent Rhinitis: There Is No Significant Difference Between Antibiotics." *BMJ* 333, no. 7564 (2006): 395; author reply 96.

Dorsen, C. "Review: Antibiotics Are Effective for Acute Purulent Rhinitis but Are Associated with Increased Gastrointestinal Side Effects." *Evid Based Nurs* 10, no. 1 (2007): 9.

Friedman, R. "Antibiotics and Acute Purulent Rhinitis: Review Is Symptomatic of Medicine Today." *BMJ* 333, no. 7564 (2006): 396; author reply 96.

Mant, A. "Does Green Snot Mean You Need Antibiotics?" ABC Health & Wellbeing, http://www.abc.net.au/health/talkinghealth/factbuster/stories/2008/02/06/2153209.htm.

O'Connor, A. "The Claim: With a Runny Nose, Green Calls for an Antibiotic." *New York Times*, 6 October 2009.

Rimmer, J., and J. Almeyda. "Antibiotics and Acute Purulent Rhinitis: Are Antibiotics Effective for Acute Purulent Rhinitis?" *BMJ* 333, no. 7564 (2006): 395–6; author reply 96.

Ross, V. "What Makes Snot Turn Green?" Scienceline (2010), http://www.scienceline.org/2010/02/01/what-makes-snot-turn-green/.

Women do not have a G-spot

Hines, T. M. "The G-Spot: A Modern Gynecologic Myth." *Am J Obstet Gynecol* 185, no. 2 (2001): 359–62.

Jannini, E. A., B. Whipple, S. A. Kingsberg, O. Buisson, P. Foldes, and Y. Vardi. "Who's Afraid of the G-Spot?" *J Sex Med* 7, no. 1, pt 1: 25–34, 2010.

Pastor, Z. "G Spot—Myths and Reality." *Ceska Gynekol* 75, no. 3: 211–7, 2010.

Roberts, Y. "The Real G-spot Myth" guardian.uk. (2010), http://www.guardian.co.uk/commentisfree/2010/jan/05/g-spot-women-study. (Accessed 10/7/10.)

Stanglin, D. "British Team Says Elusive G-spot May Be a Myth." USAToday.com (2010), content.usatoday.com/communities/ondeadline/post/2010/01/british-team-says-elusive-g-spot-may-be-a-myth/1. (Accessed 10/7/10.)

Zaviacic, M., and R. J. Ablin. "The G-Spot." *Am J Obstet Gynecol* 187, no. 2 (2002): 519–20; discusssion 20.

Dyeing your hair will give your baby birth defects

Burnett, C., E. I. Goldenthal, S. B. Harris, F. X. Wazeter, J. Strausburg, R. Kapp, and R. Voelker. "Teratology and Percutaneous Toxicity Studies on Hair Dyes." *J Toxicol Environ Health* 1, no. 6 (1976): 1027–40.

Burnett, C., R. Loehr, and J. Corbett. "Heritable Translocation Study on Two Hair Dye Formulations." *Fundam Appl Toxicol* 1, no. 4 (1981): 325–8.

DiNardo, J. C., J. C. Picciano, R. W. Schnetzinger, W. E. Morris, and B. A. Wolf. "Teratological Assessment of Five Oxidative Hair Dyes in the Rat." *Toxicol Appl Pharmacol* 78, no. 1 (1985): 163–6.

"Hair Dye FAQs." WebMD.com, http://www.webmd.com/skin-beauty/hair-dye-faqs?page=2.

"Hair Dyes." American Cancer Society, http://www.cancer.org/Cancer/CancerCauses/OtherCarcinogens/IntheWorkplace/hair-dyes. (Accessed 8/5/10.)

Harms, R. "Hair Dye and Pregnancy: A Concern?" MayoClinic.com, http://www.mayoclinic.com/health/hair-dye-and-pregnancy/AN00241. (Accessed 7/1/10).

McCall, E. E., A. F. Olshan, and J. L. Daniels. "Maternal Hair Dye Use and Risk of Neuroblastoma in Offspring." *Cancer Causes Control* 16, no. 6 (2005): 743–8.

Don't shake hands if you want to stay healthy

Arold, E. "Should You Stop Shaking Hands During This Flu Season?" Helium .com. (Accessed 6/29/10.)

Bouchez, C. "Presidential Advice: Shake Off a Cold." WebMD, http://www.medicinenet.com/script/main/art.asp?articlekey=50382. (Accessed 6/29/10.)

"Prevent Colds with Hand Washing." WebMD, http://www.webmd.com/cold-and-flu/cold-guide/cold-prevention-hand-washing. (Accessed 6/30/10.)

Royle, J. R. "With Swine Flu on the Rise, Should We Stop Shaking Hands?" (2009), http://www.foxnews.com/story/0,2933,518387,00.html.

Saether, L. "Cold Season Question: To Shake or Not to Shake?" CNNhealth .com (2007), http://www.cnn.com/2007/HEALTH/12/28/hfh.germs/index.html.

You shouldn't enter the home of someone who is sick

Cowling, B. J., R. O. Fung, C. K. Cheng, V. J. Fang, K. H. Chan, W. H. Seto, R. Yung, B. Chiu, P. Lee, T. M. Uyeki, P. M. Houck, J. S. Peiris, and G. M. Leung. "Preliminary Findings of a Randomized Trial of Non-Pharmaceutical Interventions to Prevent Influenza Transmission in Households." *PLoS One* 3, no. 5 (2008): e2101.

Dennehy, P. H. "Transmission of Rotavirus and Other Enteric Pathogens in the Home." *Pediatr Infect Dis J* 19, no. 10 Suppl (2000): S103–5.

Goldmann, D. A. "Transmission of Viral Respiratory Infections in the Home." *Pediatr Infect Dis J* 19, no. 10 Suppl (2000): S97–102.

"How the Flu Spreads." CDC.com, http://www.cdc.gov/flu/about/disease/spread.htm, 2010. (Accessed 6/2/10.)

Larson, E. L. "Warned, but Not Well Armed: Preventing Viral Upper Respiratory Infections in Households." *Public Health Nurs* 24, no. 1 (2007): 48–59.

Larson, E. L., Y. H. Ferng, J. Wong-McLoughlin, S. Wang, M. Haber, and S. S. Morse. "Impact of Non-Pharmaceutical Interventions on Uris and Influenza in Crowded, Urban Households." *Public Health Rep* 125, no. 2 (2010): 178–91.

Samet, J. M. "How Do We Catch Colds?" *Am J Respir Crit Care Med* 169, no. 11 (2004): 1175–6.

I have just the thing for that cold . . . Honey and Vinegar

"Cough and Cold Remedies for the Treatment of Acute Respiratory Infections in Young Children." Department of Child and Adolescent Health, World Health Organization, Geneva, 2001.

Dealleaume, L., B. Tweed, and J. O. Neher. "Do OTC Remedies Relieve Cough in Acute Upper Respiratory Infections?" *J Fam Pract* 58, no. 10 (2009): 559a–c.

Moyad, M. A. "Conventional and Alternative Medical Advice for Cold and Flu Prevention: What Should Be Recommended and What Should Be Avoided?" *Urol Nurs* 29, no. 6 (2009): 455–8.

Paul, I. M., J. Beiler, A. McMonagle, M. L. Shaffer, L. Duda, and C. M. Berlin, Jr. "Effect of Honey, Dextromethorphan, and No Treatment on Nocturnal Cough and Sleep Quality for Coughing Children and Their Parents." *Arch Pediatr Adolesc Med* 161, no. 12 (2007): 1140–6.

Pourahmad, M., and S. Sobhanian. "Effect of Honey on the Common Cold." *Arch Med Res* 40, no. 3 (2009): 224–5.

Eating local honey will prevent allergies

Clark, J. "Can You Fight Allergies with Local Honey?" Discovery Health, http://health.howstuffworks.com/diseases-conditions/allergies/local-honey-for-allergies.htm.

Foreman, J. "Does Eating 'Local Honey' Help Prevent Allergies?" *Boston Globe* (2008), http://www.boston.com/news/science/articles/2008/06/23/does_eating_local_honey_help_prevent_allergies/.

"Honey Effective in Killing Bacteria That Cause Chronic Sinusitis." *Science-Daily* (2008), http://www.sciencedaily.com/releases/2008/09/080923091335.htm.

Ishikawa, Y., T. Tokura, N. Nakano, M. Hara, F. Niyonsaba, H. Ushio, Y. Yamamoto, T. Tadokoro, K. Okumura, and H. Ogawa. "Inhibitory Effect of Honeybee-Collected Pollen on Mast Cell Degranulation in Vivo and in Vitro." *J Med Food* 11, no. 1 (2008): 14–20.

Knox, A. "Harnessing Honey's Healing Power." BBC News (2004), http://news.bbc.co.uk/2/hi/health/3787867.stm.

Opar, A. "Does Eating Local Honey Help Prevent Allergies?" Audubonmagazine.org, http://magblog.audubon.org/does-eating-local-honey-help-prevent-allergies.

Simon, A., K. Traynor, K. Santos, G. Blaser, U. Bode, and P. Molan. "Medical Honey for Wound Care—Still the 'Latest Resort'?" *Evid Based Complement Alternat Med* 6, no. 2 (2009): 165–73.

Hot peppers can cause ulcers

Abdel-Salam, O. M., J. Szolcsanyi, and G. Mozsik. "Capsaicin and the Stomach. A Review of Experimental and Clinical Data." *J Physiol Paris* 91, no. 3–5 (1997): 151–71. http://www.fitsugar.com/Hot-Pepper-Nasal-Spray—-Would-You-Try-251471

"Hot Pepper Nasal Spray—Would You Try It?" FitSugar.com, http://www.fitsugar.com/Hot-Pepper-Nasal-Spray—-Would-You-Try-251471.

"Hot Pepper Treat Pancreatic Cancer." In *Foods That Heal*, 2006. http://foodheal.blogspot.com/2006/04/hot-pepper-treat-pancreatic-cancer_23.html

Mozsik, G., A. Vincze, and J. Szolcsanyi. "Four Response Stages of Capsaicin-Sensitive Primary Afferent Neurons to Capsaicin and Its Analog: Gastric Acid Secretion, Gastric Mucosal Damage and Protection." *J Gastroenterol Hepatol* 16, no. 10 (2001): 1093–7.

Parker-Pope, T. "Hillary's Health Plan: Hot Peppers." In *Well*. New York City: The New York Times Company, 2008. http://well.blogs.nytimes.com/2008/02/12/hillarys-health-plan-hot-peppers.

Satyanarayana, M. N. "Capsaicin and Gastric Ulcers." *Crit Rev Food Sci Nutr* 46, no. 4 (2006): 275–328.

Swan, D. "Peppers Are Hot—As a Health and Diet Aid." *Medill Reports* (2006), http://news.medill.northwestern.edu/chicago/news.aspx?id=62587.

Szolcsanyi, J., and L. Bartho. "Capsaicin-Sensitive Afferents and Their Role in Gastroprotection: An Update." *J Physiol Paris* 95, no. 1–6 (2001): 181–8.

Teng, C. H., J. Y. Kang, A. Wee, and K. O. Lee. "Protective Action of Capsaicin and Chilli on Haemorrhagic Shock-Induced Gastric Mucosal Injury in the Rat." *J Gastroenterol Hepatol* 13, no. 10 (1998): 1007–14.

Hydrogen peroxide is good for a wound

Beattie, C., L. E. Harry, S. A. Hamilton, and D. Burke. "Cardiac Arrest Following Hydrogen Peroxide Irrigation of a Breast Wound." *J Plast Reconstr Aesthet Surg* 63, no. 3 (2010): e253–4.

Curtis, P. "7 First-Aid Standbys You Should Never Use." *Reader's Digest*, October 2004, http://www.rd.com/living-healthy/7-first-aid-standbys-you-should-never-use/article14315.html.

O'Connor, A. "The Claim: Hydrogen Peroxide Is a Good Treatment for Small Wounds." *New York Times* (2007), http://www.nytimes.com/2007/06/19/health/19real.html.

Thomas, G. W., L. T. Rael, R. Bar-Or, R. Shimonkevitz, C. W. Mains, D. S. Slone, M. L. Craun, and D. Bar-Or. "Mechanisms of Delayed Wound Healing by Commonly Used Antiseptics." *J Trauma* 66, no. 1 (2009): 82–90; discussion 90–1.

Torres, J. "Hydrogen Peroxide for Wound Cleaning: Water's Better!" My Family Doctor, http://familydoctormag.com/first-aid-and-safety/1361-hydrogen-peroxide-for-wounds-is-it-better-than-water.html.

If you cut off your finger, put it on ice right away

"Amputation—Traumatic." NYTimes.com, http://health.nytimes.com/health/guides/injury/amputation-traumatic/overview.html. (Accessed 7/8/10.)

Engber, D. "Doctor, Please Reattach My . . ." *Slate* (2005), http://www.slate.com/id/2113866.

Kaplan, J. "Severed or Constricted Limbs or Digits." Merck, http://www.merck.com/mmhe/sec24/ch299/ch299h.html.

Langdorf, M. "Replantation: Treatment and Medication." eMedicine, http://emedicine.medscape.com/article/827648-treatment.

"Severed Fingers." Editorial, *Br Med J* 2, no. 5914 (1974): 291.

"Severed Penis Retrieved from Toilet Is Reattached." Reuters (2005), http://forums.canadiancontent.net/535707-post1.html.

Scaletta, T. "Top 10 First Aid Mistakes." *Newsweek* (2008), http://www.newsweek.com/2008/04/13/top-10-first-aid-mistakes.html. (Accessed 7/8/10.)

If you catch a cold, it means you have a weak immune system

Cohen, S., W. J. Doyle, C. M. Alper, D. Janicki-Deverts, and R. B. Turner. "Sleep Habits and Susceptibility to the Common Cold." *Arch Intern Med* 169, no. 1 (2009): 62–7.

Cohen, S., W. J. Doyle, D. P. Skoner, B. S. Rabin, and J. M. Gwaltney, Jr. "Social Ties and Susceptibility to the Common Cold." *JAMA* 277, no. 24 (1997): 1940–4.

Cohen, S., D. A. Tyrrell, M. A. Russell, M. J. Jarvis, and A. P. Smith. "Smoking, Alcohol Consumption, and Susceptibility to the Common Cold." *Am J Public Health* 83, no. 9 (1993): 1277–83.

Cohen, S., D. A. Tyrrell, and A. P. Smith. "Psychological Stress and Susceptibility to the Common Cold." *N Engl J Med* 325, no. 9 (1991): 606–12.

Gwaltney, J. M., Jr., and F. G. Hayden. "Myths of the Common Cold." http://www.commoncold.org/special1.htm. (Accessed 6/9/10.)

Gwaltney, J. M., Jr., J. O. Hendley, G. Simon, and W. S. Jordan, Jr. "Rhinovirus Infections in an Industrial Population. II. Characteristics of Illness and Antibody Response." *JAMA* 202, no. 6 (1967): 494–500.

You can only get lice from another person with lice

Burkhart, C. N. "Fomite Transmission with Head Lice: A Continuing Controversy." *Lancet* 361, no. 9352 (2003): 99–100.

Burkhart, C. N., and C. G. Burkhart. "Fomite Transmission in Head Lice." *J Am Acad Dermatol* 56, no. 6 (2007): 1044–7.

Canyon, D., and R. Speare. "Do Head Lice Spread in Swimming Pools?" *Int J Dermatol* 46, no. 11 (2007): 1211–3.

"Head Lice." *Paediatr Child Health* 13, no. 8 (2008): 697–706.

"Head Lice." Baltimore County Department of Health, http://www.baltimorecountymd.gov/Agencies/health/healthservices/children/headlice.html. (Accessed 6/29/10.)

Sciscione, P., and C. A. Krause-Parello. "No-Nit Policies in Schools: Time for Change." *J Sch Nurs* 23, no. 1 (2007): 13–20.

Speare, R., C. Cahill, and G. Thomas. "Head Lice on Pillows, and Strategies to Make a Small Risk Even Less." *Int J Dermatol* 42, no. 8 (2003): 626–9.

Takano-Lee, M., J. D. Edman, B. A. Mullens, and J. M. Clark. "Transmission Potential of the Human Head Louse, Pediculus Capitis (Anoplura: Pediculidae)." *Int J Dermatol* 44, no. 10 (2005): 811–6.

Marriage makes you healthy

Bennett, K. M. "Does Marital Status and Marital Status Change Predict Physical Health in Older Adults?" *Psychol Med* 36, no. 9 (2006): 1313–20.

Manzoli, L., P. Villari, M. Pirone G, and A. Boccia. "Marital Status and Mortality in the Elderly: A Systematic Review and Meta-Analysis." *Soc Sci Med* 64, no. 1 (2007): 77–94.

Parker-Pope, T. "Is Marriage Good for Your Health?" NYTimes.com (2010), http://www.nytimes.com/2010/04/18/magazine/18marriage-t.html. (Accessed 10/7/10.)

Pinsof, W. M. "The Death of 'Till Death Us Do Part': The Transformation of Pair-Bonding in the 20th Century." *Fam Process* 41, no. 2 (2002): 135–57.

Umberson, D., K. Williams, D. A. Powers, H. Liu, and B. Needham. "You Make Me Sick: Marital Quality and Health over the Life Course." *J Health Soc Behav* 47, no. 1 (2006): 1–16.

Masturbation will make you go blind

Ashworth, M. "Do Kellogg's Corn Flakes Help Control Masturbation?" Psych-Central, http://psychcentral.com/lib/2007/do-kelloggs-corn-flakes-help-control-masturbation/. (Accessed 6/29/10.)

———. "Does Masturbation Cause Blindness?" PsychCentral, http://psych central.com/lib/2007/does-masturbation-cause-blindness/. (Accessed 6/29/10.)

Auteri, S. "5 Bogus Masturbation Myths." YourTango, http://www.yourtango .com/201055179/5-bogus-masturbation-myths. (Accessed 6/29/10.)

Dr. V. "Doin' It with Dr. V: Masturbation Myths." TheFrisky, http://www.the frisky.com/post/246-doin-it-with-dr-v-masturbation-myths/. (Accessed 6/29/10.)

Macintyre, B. "Birthday of One Mighty Flake . . . And a Cereal Too." *The Times* (London) (2006), http://www.timesonline.co.uk/tol/news/world/us_and_ameri-cas/article732027.ece. (Accessed 6/29/10.)

Shaw, J. "Masturbation Myths." 4-Men.org, http://www.4-men.org/myths-about-masturbation.html. (Accessed 6/29/10.)

Silverberg, C. "100 Years of Fighting Masturbation, One Spoonful at a Time." About.com, http://sexuality.about.com/b/2006/02/20/100-years-of-fighting-mas turbation-one-spoonful-at-a-time.htm. (Accessed 6/29/10.)

Witmer, D. "Masturbation Myths." About.com, http://parentingteens.about. com/od/masterbationmyths/a/masterbation.htm. (Accessed 6/29/10.)

Your amalgam or metal fillings will make you sick

"About Dental Amalgam Fillings." U.S. Food and Drug Administration (FDA), http://www.fda.gov/MedicalDevices/ProductsandMedicalProcedures/Dental Products/DentalAmalgam/ucm171094.htm#3. (Accessed 6/16/10.)

Edlich, R. F., C. L. Cross, C. A. Wack, W. B. Long III, and A. T. Newkirk. "The Food and Drug Administration Agrees to Classify Mercury Fillings." *J Environ Pathol Toxicol Oncol* 27, no. 4 (2008): 303–5.

Gardner, R. M., J. F. Nyland, I. A. Silva, A. M. Ventura, J. M. de Souza, and E. K. Silbergeld. "Mercury Exposure, Serum Antinuclear/Antinucleolar Antibodies, and Serum Cytokine Levels in Mining Populations in Amazonian Brazil: A Cross-Sectional Study." *Environ Res* 110, no. 4 (2010): 345–54.

Magruder, M. "Mercury Amalgam Fillings Issue Continues to Generate Controversy." *Malibu Times*, 3 September 2008.

McGrath, Peta. "Sick to the Back Teeth." *The Guardian* (London), 23 November 2004.

Weidenhammer, W., C. Hausteiner, T. Zilker, D. Melchart, and S. Bornschein. "Does a Specific Dental Amalgam Syndrome Exist? A Comparative Study." *Acta Odontol Scand* (2009): 1–7.

Wojcik, D. P., M. E. Godfrey, D. Christie, and B. E. Haley. "Mercury Toxicity Presenting as Chronic Fatigue, Memory Impairment and Depression: Diagnosis, Treatment, Susceptibility, and Outcomes in a New Zealand General Practice Setting (1994–2006)." *Neuro Endocrinol Lett* 27, no. 4 (2006): 415–23.

Eating fish while you are pregnant will give your baby birth defects

Davidson, P. W., G. J. Myers, and B. Weiss. "Mercury Exposure and Child Development Outcomes." *Pediatrics* 113, no. 4 Suppl (2004): 1023–9.

"Foods to Avoid During Pregnancy." American Pregnancy Association, http://www.americanpregnancy.org/pregnancyhealth/foodstoavoid.html. (Accessed 7/1/10.)

"General Information on the Risk of Eating Fish." Texas Department of State Health Services, http://www.dshs.state.tx.us/seafood/eatrisk.shtm. (Accessed 7/1/10.)

Mozaffarian, D., and E. B. Rimm. "Fish Intake, Contaminants, and Human Health: Evaluating the Risks and the Benefits." *JAMA* 296, no. 15 (2006): 1885–99.

U.S. Department of Health & Human Services. "What to Eat While Pregnant." WomensHealth.gov, http://www.womenshealth.gov/Pregnancy/pregnancy/eat.cfm#fish. (Accessed 7/1/10.)

A glass of warm milk will put you to sleep

Ancoli-Israel, S. " 'Sleep Is Not Tangible' Or What the Hebrew Tradition Has to Say About Sleep." *Psychosom Med* 63, no. 5 (2001): 778–87.

Consumer Guide. "26 Home Remedies for Insomnia." DiscoveryHealth.com, http://health.howstuffworks.com/wellness/natural-medicine/home-remedies/home-remedies-for-insomnia2.htm. (Accessed 7/7/10.)

Hudson, C., S. P. Hudson, T. Hecht, and J. MacKenzie. "Protein Source Tryptophan Versus Pharmaceutical Grade Tryptophan as an Efficacious Treatment for Chronic Insomnia." *Nutr Neurosci* 8, no. 2 (2005): 121–7.

Markus, C. R., C. Firk, C. Gerhardt, J. Kloek, and G. F. Smolders. "Effect of Different Tryptophan Sources on Amino Acids Availability to the Brain and Mood in Healthy Volunteers." *Psychopharmacology (Berl)* 201, no. 1 (2008): 107–14.

Morgenthaler, T. "Are There Any Foods That Help You Sleep Better?" MayoClinic.com. (Accessed 7/7/10.)

Morrow, J. "Insomnia Prevention and Treatment Options." OmniMedicalSearch.com, http://www.omnimedicalsearch.com/conditions-diseases/insomnia-prevention-treatment.html. (Accessed 7/7/10.)

Riemann, D., B. Feige, M. Hornyak, S. Koch, F. Hohagen, and U. Voderholzer. "The Tryptophan Depletion Test: Impact on Sleep in Primary Insomnia—A Pilot Study." *Psychiatry Res* 109, no. 2 (2002): 129–35.

Ringdahl, E. N., S. L. Pereira, and J. E. Delzell, Jr. "Treatment of Primary Insomnia." *J Am Board Fam Pract* 17, no. 3 (2004): 212–9.

Sproule, B. A., U. E. Busto, C. Buckle, N. Herrmann, and S. Bowles. "The Use of Non-Prescription Sleep Products in the Elderly." *Int J Geriatr Psychiatry* 14, no. 10 (1999): 851–7.

"Which Technique Is Best for Treating Insomnia?" NineMSN.com, http://health.ninemsn.com.au/whatsgoodforyou/theshow/693990/which-technique-is-best-for-treating-insomnia. (Accessed 7/7/10.)

I have just the thing for that cold . . . Neti Pots

Kassel, J. C., D. King, and G. K. Spurling. "Saline Nasal Irrigation for Acute Upper Respiratory Tract Infections." *Cochrane Database Syst Rev* 3 (2010): CD006821. (Accessed 8/4/10.)

Oz, M. "The Best of Dr. Oz." Oprah.com, http://www.oprah.com/health/Best-of-Dr-Oz-5-Years-of-Memorable-Moments/18. (Accessed 8/4/10.)

————. "Your Questions Answered." Oprah.com, http://www.oprah.com/health/Your-Questions-Answered/6.

Rabago, D., B. Barrett, L. Marchand, R. Maberry, and M. Mundt. "Qualitative Aspects of Nasal Irrigation Use by Patients with Chronic Sinus Disease in a Multimethod Study." *Ann Fam Med* 4, no. 4 (2006): 295–301.

Rabago, D., T. Pasic, A. Zgierska, M. Mundt, B. Barrett, and R. Maberry. "The Efficacy of Hypertonic Saline Nasal Irrigation for Chronic Sinonasal Symptoms." *Otolaryngol Head Neck Surg* 133, no. 1 (2005): 3–8.

Rabago, D., and A. Zgierska. "Saline Nasal Irrigation for Upper Respiratory Conditions." *Am Fam Physician* 80, no. 10 (2009): 1117–9.

Rabago, D., A. Zgierska, M. Mundt, B. Barrett, J. Bobula, and R. Maberry. "Efficacy of Daily Hypertonic Saline Nasal Irrigation Among Patients with Sinusitis: A Randomized Controlled Trial." *J Fam Pract* 51, no. 12 (2002): 1049–55.

Tilt your head back to stop a nosebleed

Brouhard, R. "How to Stop a Bloody Nose." About.com, http://firstaid.about.com/od/bleedingcontrol/ht/06_epistaxis.htm. (Accessed 7/17/10.)

Davidson, T. M., and D. Davidson. "Immediate Management of Epistaxis: Bloody Nuisance or Ominous Sign?" *Phys Sportsmed* 24, no. 8 (1996): 74–83.

Dowshen, S. "Nosebleeds." KidsHealth.org, http://kidshealth.org/teen/safety/first_aid/nosebleeds.html#. (Accessed 7/7/10.)

Lyden, J. "Stopping Nose Bleeds." http://childcarebyjudylyden.blogspot.com/2007/05/stopping-nose-bleeds.html. (Accessed 7/7/10.)

O'Connor, A. "The Claim: Tilt Your Head Back to Treat a Nosebleed." *New York Times* (2008), http://www.nytimes.com/2008/04/29/health/29real.html?em&ex=1209873600&en=b5b0127505962f5e&ei=5087%0A.

You can't get a sexually transmitted disease from oral sex

"HIV Transmission." Centers for Disease Control and Prevention, http://www.cdc.gov/hiv/resources/qa/transmission.htm. (Accessed 6/29/10.)

"Hotline: Can You Get an STD from Oral Sex?" Stdtestexpress, http://www.stdtestexpress.com/blog/2009/11/hotline-can-you-get-an-std-from-oral-sex/. (Accessed 6/29/10.)

Peiperl, L. "Frequently Asked Questions." Department of Veterans Affairs, http://www.hiv.va.gov/vahiv?page=ptfaq-2006-02-27. (Accessed 6/29/10.)

"Q&A/Articles." TeenGrowth.com, http://www.teengrowth.com/index.cfm?action=info_advice&ID_Advice=2454. (Accessed 6/29/10.)

Oysters are an aphrodisiac

"Are Oysters Really Aphrodisiacs." (2010), http://www.sixwise.com/newsletters/06/02/16/are-oysters-really-aphrodisiacs.htm. (Accessed 10/6/10.)

McNeil, S. "Aphrodisiac Foods: Fact or Fiction?" (2010), http://www.askmen.com/sports/foodcourt/56_eating_well.html. (Accessed 10/6/10.)

Men's Health News. "Are Oysters Really Aphrodisiacs." (2010), http://www.medindia.net/news/view_news_main.asp?x=18460. (Accessed 10/6/10.)

"Pearly Wisdom: Oysters Are an Aphrodisiac" *Sydney Morning Herald* (2010), http://www.smh.com.au/articles/2005/03/23/1111525227607.html. (Accessed 10/6/10.)

Shulman, M. "The Science of Aphrodisiacs" U.S. News & World Report (2010), http://health.usnews.com/health-news/familyhealth/sexual-and-reproductive-health/articles/2008/08/19/the-science-of-aphrodisiacs.html. (Accessed 10/6/10.)

Sinclair Intimacy Institute. "Aphrodisiacs." Discovery Health (2010), http://healthguide.howstuffworks.com/aphrodisiacs-dictionary1.htm. (Accessed 10/6/10.)

"Top 10 Aphrodisiacs." LiveScience.com. (2010), http://www.livescience.com/health/top10_aphrodisiacs-1.html. (Accessed 10/6/10.)

You can make your penis bigger without surgery

Aghamir, M. K., R. Hosseini, and F. Alizadeh. "A Vacuum Device for Penile Elongation: Fact or Fiction?" *BJU Int* 97, no. 4 (2006): 777–8.

Kwak, T. I., M. Oh, J. J. Kim, and D. G. Moon. "The Effects of Penile Girth Enhancement Using Injectable Hyaluronic Acid Gel, a Filler." *J Sex Med* (March 11, 2010).

"Penis-Enlargement Scams: You're More Normal than You Think." MayoClinic.com (2010), http://www.mayoclinic.com/health/penis/MC00026.

Marks, S. "Penis Enlargement: Myths and Facts." WebMD.com (2010), http://blogs.webmd.com/mens-health-office/2008/04/penis-enlargement-myths-and-facts.html. (Accessed 10/7/10.)

Nikoobakht, M., A. Shahnazari, M. Rezaeidanesh, A. Mehrsai, and G. Pourmand. "Effect of Penile-Extender Device in Increasing Penile Size in Men with Shortened Penis: Preliminary Results." *J Sex Med* (Jan. 19, 2010).

Nugteren, H. M., G. T. Balkema, A. L. Pascal, W. C. Schultz, J. M. Nijman, and M. F. van Driel. "Penile Enlargement: From Medication to Surgery." *J Sex Marital Ther* 36, no. 2: 118–23.

Park, S. W., C. H. Lee, D. H. Shin, N. S. Bang, and S. M. Lee. "Effect of Sa1, a Herbal Formulation, on Sexual Behavior and Penile Erection." *Biol Pharm Bull* 29, no. 7 (2006): 1383–6.

"Penis Myths Debunked." LiveScience.com (2010), http://www.livescience.com/health/070601_penis_myths.html. (Accessed 10/7/10.)

Vardi, Y., Y. Har-Shai, T. Gil, and I. Gruenwald. "A Critical Analysis of Penile Enhancement Procedures for Patients with Normal Penile Size: Surgical Techniques, Success, and Complications." *Eur Urol* 54, no. 5 (2008): 1042–50.

If you swallow something poisonous, you need to vomit as soon as possible

Bond, G. R. "Home Syrup of Ipecac Use Does Not Reduce Emergency Department Use or Improve Outcome." *Pediatrics* 112, no. 5 (2003): 1061–4.

"Drain Cleaners." NYTimes.com, http://health.nytimes.com/health/guides/poison/drain-cleaners/overview.html. (Accessed 7/8/10.)

"Poison First Aid: What to Do if Poisoned." Minnesota Poison Control, http://www.mnpoison.org/index.asp?pageID=49. (Accessed 7/8/10.)

"Poisoning: When to Induce Vomiting." FamilyEducation.com, http://life.familyeducation.com/first-aid/poisons/48282.html. (Accessed 7/8/10.)

"Position Paper: Ipecac Syrup." *J Toxicol Clin Toxicol* 42, no. 2 (2004): 133–43.

"Throw Out Syrup of Ipecac." Yale-New Haven Children's Hospital, http://www.ynhh.org/healthlink/pediatrics/pediatrics_2_04.html. (Accessed 7/8/10.)

"Vomiting—First Aid for Poisoning? An Incorrect Assumption." New Zealand National Poisons Centre, http://poisons.co.nz/fact.php?f=19. (Accessed 7/8/10.)

Eating extra protein after you work out will help you build muscles

Cribb, P. J., A. D. Williams, M. F. Carey, and A. Hayes. "The Effect of Whey Isolate and Resistance Training on Strength, Body Composition, and Plasma Glutamine." *Int J Sport Nutr Exerc Metab* 16, no. 5 (2006): 494–509.

Hulmi, J. J., V. Kovanen, H. Selanne, W. J. Kraemer, K. Hakkinen, and A. A. Mero. "Acute and Long-Term Effects of Resistance Exercise with or Without Protein Ingestion on Muscle Hypertrophy and Gene Expression." *Amino Acids* 37, no. 2 (2009): 297–308.

Kerksick, C. M., C. Rasmussen, S. Lancaster, M. Starks, P. Smith, C. Melton, M. Greenwood, A. Almada, and R. Kreider. "Impact of Differing Protein Sources and a Creatine Containing Nutritional Formula after 12 Weeks of Resistance Training." *Nutrition* 23, no. 9 (2007): 647–56.

Osterweil, N. "The Benefits of Protein." WebMD.com (2010), http://www.webmd.com/fitness-exercise/guide/benefits-protein. (Accessed 10/7/10.)

Phillips, S. M., J. E. Tang, and D. R. Moore. "The Role of Milk- and Soy-Based Protein in Support of Muscle Protein Synthesis and Muscle Protein Accretion in Young and Elderly Persons." *J Am Coll Nutr* 28, no. 4 (2009): 343–54.

Quill, S. (2010) "7 Muscle Myths." Active.com (2010), http://www.active.com/fitness/Articles/7_Muscle_Myths.htm. (Accessed 10/7/10.)

Waehner, P. "Fitness Myths—Protein, Weight Training and More." 2010, http://exercise.about.com/cs/exercisehealth/a/FitnessMyths_2.htm. (Accessed 10/7/10.)

Willoughby, D. S., J. R. Stout, and C. D. Wilborn. "Effects of Resistance Training and Protein Plus Amino Acid Supplementation on Muscle Anabolism, Mass, and Strength." *Amino Acids* 32, no. 4 (2007): 467–77.

Saunas or sweat lodges will cleanse your body of toxins

Blum, N., and A. Blum. "Beneficial Effects of Sauna Bathing for Heart Failure Patients." *Exp Clin Cardiol* 12, no. 1 (2007): 29–32.

Brandis, K. "Fluid Physiology: Sweat." http://www.anaesthesiamcq.com/Fluid Book/fl3_3.php. (Accessed 8/26/10.)

Brown, A. "Sweat Lodges and Safety." About.com, http://spas.about.com/od/spahistoryandculture/a/sweatlodgesafety.htm. (Accessed 8/26/10.)

Dougherty, J. "Deaths at Sweat Lodge Bring Soul-Searching." *New York Times* (2009), http://www.nytimes.com/2009/10/12/us/12lodge.html?_r=1. (Accessed 8/26/10.)

Eren, B., R. Fedakar, N. Turkmen, and O. Akan. "Deaths in the Turkish Hamam (Hot Bath)." *Bratisl Lek Listy* 110, no. 11 (2009): 697–700.

Hannuksela, M. L., and S. Ellahham. "Benefits and Risks of Sauna Bathing." *Am J Med* 110, no. 2 (2001): 118–26.

Kenttamies, A., and K. Karkola. "Death in Sauna." *J Forensic Sci* 53, no. 3 (2008): 724–9.

Koljonen, V. "Hot Air Sauna Burns—Review of Their Etiology and Treatment." *J Burn Care Res* 30, no. 4 (2009): 705–10.

Kukkonen-Harjula, K., and K. Kauppinen. "Health Effects and Risks of Sauna Bathing." *Int J Circumpolar Health* 65, no. 3 (2006): 195–205.

Livingston, R. "Medical Risks and Benefits of the Sweat Lodge." *J Altern Complement Med* 16, no. 6 (2010): 617–9.

Martini, F., and J. Nath. "Sebaceous Glands and Sweat Glands Are Exocrine Glands Found in the Skin." In *Fundamentals of Anatomy and Physiology*, 8th ed., 172–73: Benjamin Cummings, 2009.

Nguyen, Y., N. Naseer, and W. H. Frishman. "Sauna as a Therapeutic Option for Cardiovascular Disease." *Cardiol Rev* 12, no. 6 (2004): 321–4.

Sohn, I. S., J. M. Cho, W. S. Kim, C. J. Kim, K. S. Kim, J. H. Bae, and C. Tei. "Preliminary Clinical Experience with Waon Therapy in Korea: Safety and Effect." *J Cardiovasc Ultrasound* 18, no. 2 (2010): 37–42.

Thomas, J. "Sweat Lodges, Steam Rooms Aren't for Detox." Health.Usnews .com, http://health.usnews.com/health-news/managing-your-healthcare/articles/2010/02/12/sweat-lodges-steam-rooms-arent-for-detox.html. (Accessed 8/26/10.)

Whiteley Clinic. "Sweating." http://www.sweating.co.uk/sweating.htm. (Accessed 8/26/10.)

If someone is having a seizure, you should put something in their mouth

"Epilepsy." FamilyDoctor.org, http://familydoctor.org/online/famdocen/home/common/brain/disorders/214.html. (Accessed 7/8/10.)

"First Aid for Seizures." Epilepsy Foundation, http://www.epilepsyfoundation.org/about/firstaid/index.cfm. (Accessed 7/8/10.)

O'Hara, K. A. "First Aid for Seizures: The Importance of Education and Appropriate Response." *J Child Neurol* 22, no. 5 Suppl (2007): 30S–7S.

"What to Do If You See Someone Having a Seizure." Foundation for Better Health Care, http://www.fbhc.org/Patients/Modules/ep_ifsomeone.cfm. (Accessed 7/8/10.)

"What to Do When You Witness Someone Having a Seizure." Florida Neuro-science Center, http://www.floridaneuroscience.com/blog/what-to-do-when-you-witness-someone-having-a-seizure. (Accessed 7/8/10.)

Having sex during pregnancy will hurt the baby

Clinic, OB-GYN. "Sex During Pregnancy." edited by The Ohio State University Medical Center. Columbus: The Ohio State University Medical Center, 2008, http://medicalcenter.osu.edu/PatientEd/Materials/PDFDocs/women-in/pregnancy/sexdur.pdf.(Accessed 7/1/10).

"Sex During Pregnancy." WebMD.com, http://www.webmd.com/baby/pregnancy-sex. (Accessed 7/1/10).

"Sex During Pregnancy: What's OK, What's Not." MayoClinic.com, http://www.mayoclinic.com/health/sex-during-pregnancy/HO00140. (Accessed 7/1/10).

You should not have sex or masturbate before a big game

"Can Pre-Game Sex Help Athletes?" CollegeTimes.com (2010), http://media.www.ecollegetimes.com/media/storage/paper991/news/2008/03/13/News/CanPreGame.Sex.Help.Athletes-3268598.shtml.

Douglass, L. Pregame Sex," Letter. NYTimes.com (2010), http://query.nytimes.com/gst/fullpage.html?res=9C0CE6DD1F31F934A3575AC0A9629C8B63. (Accessed 10/7/10.)

Fischer, G. "Abstention from Sex and Other Pre Game Rituals Used by College Male Varsity Athletes," 2010, http://www.questia.com/googleScholar.qst?docId=5002239512. (Accessed 10/7/10.)

Gordon, M. "College Coaches' Attitudes Toward Pregame Sex." *J Sex Res* 24, (1988): 256–62.

Lovgren, S. "Sex and Sports: Should Athletes Abstain Before Big Events." National Geographic.com (2010), http://news.nationalgeographic.com/news/2006/02/0222_060222_sex.html. (Accessed 10/7/10.)

McGinn, D. "Go Ahead and Score: Pregame Sex Has No Effect, Doctor Says." *Globe & Mail*, 2010 http://www.theglobeandmail.com/life/health/go-ahead-and-score-pregame-sex-has-no-effect-doctor-says/article1379083/. (Accessed 10/7/10.)

"Sexual Activity and Heart Disease or Stroke." American Heart Association (2010), http://www.americanheart.org/presenter.jhtml?identifier=4714. (Accessed 10/6/10.)

Temple, J. "Pre-Game Sex: A Do or a Don't?" Kansan.com (2010), http://www.kansan.com/news/2008/jul/14/sports/. (Accessed 10/7/10.)

Sex is bad for your heart

Hall, S. A., and R. Shackelton et al. (2010). "Sexual Activity, Erectile Dysfunction, and Incident Cardiovascular Events." *Am J Cardiol* 105, no 2: 192–197.

"Having Sex Twice a Week 'reduces Chance of Heart Attack by Half'" *Telegraph.* 2010, http://www.telegraph.co.uk/health/healthnews/6950548/Having-sex-twice-a-week-reduces-chance-of-heart-attack-by-half.htm. (Accessed 10/6/10.)

"Heart Attack Survivors Fear Sex." BBCNews.com (2010), http://news.bbc.co.uk/2/hi/8696801.stm. (Accessed 10/6/10.)

Hendrick, B. "More Sex Could Mean Less Heart Risk." WebMD.com (2010), http://www.webmd.com/heart-disease/news/20100121/more-sex-could-mean-less-heart-risk. (Accessed 10/6/10.)

"Sex After a Heart Attack." WebMD.com (2010), http://www.webmd.com/heart-disease/features/sex-after-a-heart-attack. (Accessed 10/6/10.)

Silverburg, C. "Heart Attack During Sex—How Common Are Heart Attacks During Sex." 2010, http://sexuality.about.com/od/sexualhealthqanda/f/heart_attack_during_sex.htm. (Accessed 10/6/10.)

Silverburg, Cory. "Sex and Heart Disease Myths—Myths Sexual Activity and Heart Disease," 2010, http://sexuality.about.com/od/sexualhealthqanda/a/myths_about_sex_and_heart_disease_attack.htm. (Accessed 10/6/10.)

Silverburg, Cory. "Sex After a Heart Attack—Resuming Sex After a Heart Attack." 2010, http://sexuality.about.com/od/sexualhealthqanda/a/sex_after_heart_attack.htm. (Accessed 10/6/10.)

Sit-ups or crunches will flatten your stomach

Friedenreich, C. M., C. G. Woolcott, A. McTiernan, T. Terry, R. Brant, R. Ballard-Barbash, M. L. Irwin, C. A. Jones, N. F. Boyd, M. J. Yaffe, K. L. Campbell, M. L. McNeely, K. H. Karvinen, and K. S. Courneya. "Adiposity Changes After a 1-Year Aerobic Exercise Intervention Among Postmenopausal Women: A Randomized Controlled Trial." *Int J Obes* (Lond). (Sept. 7, 2010).

Green, J. S., P. R. Stanforth, T. Rankinen, A. S. Leon, D. Rao Dc, J. S. Skinner, C. Bouchard, and J. H. Wilmore. "The Effects of Exercise Training on Abdominal Visceral Fat, Body Composition, and Indicators of the Metabolic Syndrome in Postmenopausal Women with and Without Estrogen Replacement Therapy: The Heritage Family Study." *Metabolism* 53, no. 9 (2004): 1192–6.

Grisaffi, D. "Abdominal Exercise Myths." 2010, http://www.flattenyourabs.net/abdominal_workout_myths.html. (Accessed 10/7/10.)

Irving, B. A., C. K. Davis, D. W. Brock, J. Y. Weltman, D. Swift, E. J. Barrett, G. A. Gaesser, and A. Weltman. "Effect of Exercise Training Intensity on Abdominal Visceral Fat and Body Composition." *Med Sci Sports Exerc* 40, no. 11 (2008): 1863–72.

Kwon, H. R., K. A. Han, Y. H. Ku, H. J. Ahn, B. K. Koo, H. C. Kim, and K. W. Min. "The Effects of Resistance Training on Muscle and Body Fat Mass and Muscle Strength in Type 2 Diabetic Women." *Korean Diabetes J* 34, no. 2: 101–10.

Newman, V. "Will Sit-ups Flatten Your Stomach?" 2010, http://www.examiner.com/fitness-in-colorado-springs/will-sit-ups-flatten-your-stomach. (Accessed 10/7/10.)

Nicklas, B. J., X. Wang, T. You, M. F. Lyles, J. Demons, L. Easter, M. J. Berry, L. Lenchik, and J. J. Carr. "Effect of Exercise Intensity on Abdominal Fat Loss During Calorie Restriction in Overweight and Obese Postmenopausal Women: A Randomized, Controlled Trial." *Am J Clin Nutr* 89, no. 4 (2009): 1043–52.

Tarig, N. "Flatten Your Stomach—Why Sit-ups Alone Won't Do It." 2010, http://ezinearticles.com/?Flatten-Your-Stomach—Why-Sit-Ups-Alone-Wont-Do-It&id=3722059. (Accessed 10/7/10.)

Your heart stops beating when you sneeze

Baraniuk, J. N., and D. Kim. "Nasonasal Reflexes, the Nasal Cycle, and Sneeze." *Curr Allergy Asthma Rep* 7, no. 2 (2007): 105–11.

Songu, M., and C. Cingi. "Sneeze Reflex: Facts and Fiction." *Ther Adv Respir Dis* 3, no. 3 (2009): 131–41.

Sitting in the snow will give you a urinary tract infection

Shaikh, N., and A. Hoberman. "Epidemiology and Risk Factors for Urinary Tract Infections in Children." UpToDate.com. (Accessed 8/2/10.)

Modgil, G., and A. Baverstock. "Should Bubble Baths Be Avoided in Children with Urinary Tract Infections?" *Arch Dis Child* 91, no. 10 (2006): 863–5.

"Urinary Tract Infections." KidsHealth.org, http://kidshealth.org/parent/infections/common/urinary.html#. (Accessed 8/2/10.)

"Urinary Tract Infection." MayoClinic.com, http://www.mayoclinic.com/health/urinary-tract-infection/DS00286/DSECTION=causes. (Accessed 6/9/10.)

"Urinary Tract Infections in Adults." National Kidney and Urologic Diseases Information Clearinghouse. http://kidney.niddk.nih.gov/kudiseases/pubs/utiadult/. (Accessed 6/9/10.)

Using soap is the best way to clean your hands

Afolabi, B. A., O. O. Oduyebo, and F. T. Ogunsola. "Bacterial Flora of Commonly Used Soaps in Three Hospitals in Nigeria." *East Afr Med J* 84, no. 10 (2007): 489–95.

Farrington, R. M., J. Rabindran, G. Crocker, R. Ali, N. Pollard, and H. R. Dalton. "'Bare Below the Elbows' and Quality of Hand Washing: A Randomised Comparison Study." *J Hosp Infect* 74, no. 1 (2010): 86–8.

Fuls, J. L., N. D. Rodgers, G. E. Fischler, J. M. Howard, M. Patel, P. L. Weidner, and M. H. Duran. "Alternative Hand Contamination Technique to Compare the Activities of Antimicrobial and Nonantimicrobial Soaps under Different Test Conditions." *Appl Environ Microbiol* 74, no. 12 (2008): 3739–44.

"Hand Washing: Do's and Don'ts." MayoClinic.com, http://www.mayoclinic.com/health/hand-washing/HQ00407. (Accessed 8/4/10.)

Hegde, P. P., A. T. Andrade, and K. Bhat. "Microbial Contamination of 'In Use' Bar Soap in Dental Clinics." *Indian J Dent Res* 17, no. 2 (2006): 70–3.

Holton, R. H., M. A. Huber, and G. T. Terezhalmy. "Antimicrobial Efficacy of Soap and Water Hand Washing Versus an Alcohol-Based Hand Cleanser." *Tex Dent J* 126, no. 12 (2009): 1175–80.

Huber, M. A., R. H. Holton, and G. T. Terezhalmy. "Cost Analysis of Hand Hygiene Using Antimicrobial Soap and Water Versus an Alcohol-Based Hand Rub." *J Contemp Dent Pract* 7, no. 2 (2006): 37–45.

Mani, A., A. M. Shubangi, and R. Saini. "Hand Hygiene Among Health Care Workers." *Indian J Dent Res* 21, no. 1 (2010): 115–8.

Manning, M. L., L. K. Archibald, L. M. Bell, S. N. Banerjee, and W. R. Jarvis. "Serratia Marcescens Transmission in a Pediatric Intensive Care Unit: A Multifactorial Occurrence." *Am J Infect Control* 29, no. 2 (2001): 115–9.

O'Connor, A. "The Claim: Always Wash Your Hands with Hot Water, Not Cold." *New York Times* (2009), http://www.nytimes.com/2009/10/13/health/13real.html?_r=1.

Pickering, A. J., A. B. Boehm, M. Mwanjali, and J. Davis. "Efficacy of Waterless Hand Hygiene Compared with Handwashing with Soap: A Field Study in Dar Es Salaam, Tanzania." *Am J Trop Med Hyg* 82, no. 2 (2010): 270–8.

Pottinger, J., S. Burns, and C. Manske. "Bacterial Carriage by Artificial Versus Natural Nails." *Am J Infect Control* 17, no. 6 (1989): 340–4.

Rabier, V., S. Bataillon, A. Jolivet-Gougeon, J. M. Chapplain, A. Beuchee, and P. Betremieux. "Hand Washing Soap as a Source of Neonatal Serratia Marcescens Outbreak." *Acta Paediatr* 97, no. 10 (2008): 1381–5.

Sartor, C., V. Jacomo, C. Duvivier, H. Tissot-Dupont, R. Sambuc, and M. Drancourt. "Nosocomial Serratia Marcescens Infections Associated with Extrinsic Contamination of a Liquid Nonmedicated Soap." *Infect Control Hosp Epidemiol* 21, no. 3 (2000): 196–9.

Smith, S. M. "A Review of Hand-Washing Techniques in Primary Care and Community Settings." *J Clin Nurs* 18, no. 6 (2009): 786–90.

Turner, R. B., J. L. Fuls, and N. D. Rodgers. "Effectiveness of Hand Sanitizers with and Without Organic Acids for Removal of Rhinovirus from Hands." *Antimicrob Agents Chemother* 54, no. 3 (2010): 1363–4.

If you wait longer to start solid foods, your baby won't get as many allergies

Allcutt, C., and M. R. Sweeney. "An Exploration of Knowledge, Attitudes and Advice Given by Health Professionals to Parents in Ireland About the Introduction of Solid Foods. A Pilot Study." *BMC Public Health* 10 (2010): 201.

Anderson, J., K. Malley, and R. Snell. "Is 6 Months Still the Best for Exclusive Breastfeeding and Introduction of Solids? A Literature Review with Consideration to the Risk of the Development of Allergies." *Breastfeed Rev* 17, no. 2 (2009): 23–31.

Branum, A., and S. Lukacs. "Food Allergy Among U.S. Children: Trends in Prevalence and Hospitalizations." National Center for Health Statistics, 2008.

"Introducing Solid Foods." Babycenter.com, http://www.babycenter.com/0_introducing-solid-foods_113.bc. (Accessed 7/1/10.)

Muche-Borowski, C., M. Kopp, I. Reese, H. Sitter, T. Werfel, and T. Schafer. "Allergy Prevention." *Dtsch Arztebl Int* 106, no. 39 (2009): 625–31.

Nwaru, B. I., M. Erkkola, S. Ahonen, M. Kaila, A. M. Haapala, C. Kronberg-Kippila, R. Salmelin, R. Veijola, J. Ilonen, O. Simell, M. Knip, and S. M. Virtanen. "Age at the Introduction of Solid Foods During the First Year and Allergic Sensitization at Age 5 Years." *Pediatrics* 125, no. 1 (2010): 50–9.

Sariachvili, M., J. Droste, S. Dom, M. Wieringa, M. Hagendorens, W. Stevens, M. van Sprundel, K. Desager, and J. Weyler. "Early Exposure to Solid Foods and the Development of Eczema in Children up to 4 Years of Age." *Pediatr Allergy Immunol* 21, no. 1, pt. 1 (2010): 74–81.

"Solid Foods: How to Get Your Baby Started." MayoClinic.com, http://www
.mayoclinic.com/health/healthy-baby/PR00029. (Accessed 7/1/10.)

Tarini, B. A., A. E. Carroll, C. M. Sox, and D. A. Christakis. "Systematic Review of the Relationship Between Early Introduction of Solid Foods to Infants
and the Development of Allergic Disease." *Arch Pediatr Adolesc Med* 160, no. 5 (2006):
502–7.

Zutavern, A., I. Brockow, B. Schaaf, A. von Berg, U. Diez, M. Borte, U. Kraemer,
O. Herbarth, H. Behrendt, H. E. Wichmann, and J. Heinrich. "Timing of Solid Food
Introduction in Relation to Eczema, Asthma, Allergic Rhinitis, and Food and In-
halant Sensitization at the Age of 6 Years: Results from the Prospective Birth Cohort Study Lisa." *Pediatrics* 121, no. 1 (2008): e44–52.

Wiping everything with a sponge will keep
the bathroom or kitchen clean

Hitti, M. "Top Spots for Bacteria at Home." WebMD Health News, http://www
.webmd.com/news/20070625/top-spots-for-bacteria-at-home. (Accessed 7/1/10.)

Mann, D. "Germs in the Kitchen." WebMD, http://www.webmd.com/food-
recipes/features/germs-in-kitchen?page=2. (Accessed 7/1/10.)

Mattick, K., K. Durham, G. Domingue, F. Jorgensen, M. Sen, D. W. Schaffner,
and T. Humphrey. "The Survival of Foodborne Pathogens During Domestic
Washing-up and Subsequent Transfer onto Washing-up Sponges, Kitchen Surfaces and Food." *Int J Food Microbiol* 85, no. 3 (2003): 213–26.

Ojima, M., Y. Toshima, E. Koya, K. Ara, H. Tokuda, S. Kawai, F. Kasuga, and N.
Ueda. "Hygiene Measures Considering Actual Distributions of Microorganisms
in Japanese Households." *J Appl Microbiol* 93, no. 5 (2002): 800–9.

Park, D. K., G. Bitton, and R. Melker. "Microbial Inactivation by Microwave
Radiation in the Home Environment." *J Environ Health* 69, no. 5 (2006): 17–24; quiz
39–40.

Sharma, M., J. Eastridge, and C. Mudd. "Effective Disinfection Methods of
Kitchen Sponges." 2007, http://www.ars.usda.gov/research/publications/publica
tions.htm?SEQ_NO_115=207115.

I have just the thing for that cold . . . Hot Steam

"Coughs, Colds, and Sinus Infections." AskDrSears.com, http://www.ask
drsears.com/html/11/T081000.asp. (Accessed 8/4/10.)

Forstall, G. J., M. L. Macknin, B. R. Yen-Lieberman, and S. V. Medendrop. "Effect of Inhaling Heated Vapor on Symptoms of the Common Cold." *JAMA* 271,
no. 14 (1994): 1109–11.

Macknin, M. L., S. Mathew, and S. V. Medendorp. "Effect of Inhaling Heated
Vapor on Symptoms of the Common Cold." *JAMA* 264, no. 8 (1990): 989–91.

Simasek, M., and D. A. Blandino. "Treatment of the Common Cold." *Am Fam
Physician* 75, no. 4 (2007): 515–20.

Singh, M. "Heated, Humidified Air for the Common Cold." *Cochrane Database
Syst Rev* 3 (2006): CD001728.

Stress will make you sick

Cohen, S., D. A. Tyrrell, and A. P. Smith. "Psychological Stress and Susceptibility to the Common Cold." *N Engl J Med* 325, no. 9 (1991): 606–12.

Do, J. E., S. M. Cho, S. I. In, K. Y. Lim, S. Lee, and E. S. Lee. "Psychosocial Aspects of Acne Vulgaris: A Community-Based Study with Korean Adolescents." *Ann Dermatol* 21, no. 2 (2009): 125–9.

Epel, E. S., E. H. Blackburn, J. Lin, F. S. Dhabhar, N. E. Adler, J. D. Morrow, and R. M. Cawthon. "Accelerated Telomere Shortening in Response to Life Stress." *Proc Natl Acad Sci U S A* 101, no. 49 (2004): 17312–5.

Epel, E. S., J. Lin, F. H. Wilhelm, O. M. Wolkowitz, R. Cawthon, N. E. Adler, C. Dolbier, W. B. Mendes, and E. H. Blackburn. "Cell Aging in Relation to Stress Arousal and Cardiovascular Disease Risk Factors." *Psychoneuroendocrinology* 31, no. 3 (2006): 277–87.

Ghodsi, S. Z., H. Orawa, and C. C. Zouboulis. "Prevalence, Severity, and Severity Risk Factors of Acne in High School Pupils: A Community-Based Study." *J Invest Dermatol* 129, no. 9 (2009): 2136–41.

"Health and Behavior: The Interplay of Biological, Behavioral, and Societal Influences." Committee on Health and Behavior: Research, Practice, and Policy, U.S. Institute of Medicine. (2001).

Kaszubowska, L. "Telomere Shortening and Ageing of the Immune System." *J Physiol Pharmacol* 59 Suppl 9 (2008): 169–86.

Kemeny, M. E., and M. Schedlowski. "Understanding the Interaction Between Psychosocial Stress and Immune-Related Diseases: A Stepwise Progression." *Brain Behav Immun* 21, no. 8 (2007): 1009–18.

Locke, S. E. "Stress, Adaptation, and Immunity: Studies in Humans." *Gen Hosp Psychiatry* 4, no. 1 (1982): 49–58.

Schleifer, S. J., S. E. Keller, and M. Stein. "Stress Effects on Immunity." *Psychiatr J Univ Ott* 10, no. 3 (1985): 125–31.

Smith, N. "Dangerous Stress and How to Wrangle It." CNN.com/living (2009), http://www.cnn.com/2009/LIVING/worklife/05/07/rs.managing.stress/.

Stone, A. A., D. H. Bovbjerg, J. M. Neale, A. Napoli, H. Valdimarsdottir, D. Cox, F. G. Hayden, and J. M. Gwaltney, Jr. "Development of Common Cold Symptoms Following Experimental Rhinovirus Infection Is Related to Prior Stressful Life Events." *Behav Med* 18, no. 3 (1992): 115–20.

"Stress and Your Health." U.S. Department of Health and Human Services, http://www.womenshealth.gov/faq/stress-your-health.cfm.

Wolkowitz, O. M., E. S. Epel, V. I. Reus, and S. H. Mellon. "Depression Gets Old Fast: Do Stress and Depression Accelerate Cell Aging?" *Depress Anxiety* 27, no. 4 (2010): 327–38.

Stress will give you high blood pressure

Alexander, C. N., R. H. Schneider, F. Staggers, W. Sheppard, B. M. Clayborne, M. Rainforth, J. Salerno, K. Kondwani, S. Smith, K. G. Walton, and B. Egan. "Trial of Stress Reduction for Hypertension in Older African Americans. II. Sex and Risk Subgroup Analysis." *Hypertension* 28, no. 2 (1996): 228–37.

Cheung, B. M., T. Au, S. Chan, C. Lam, Sh Lau, R. Lee, S. Lee, W. Lo, E. Sin, M. Tang, and H. Tsang. "The Relationship Between Hypertension and Anxiety or Depression in Hong Kong Chinese." *Exp Clin Cardiol* 10, no. 1 (2005): 21–4.

Hildrum, B., A. Mykletun, J. Holmen, and A. A. Dahl. "Effect of Anxiety and Depression on Blood Pressure: 11-Year Longitudinal Population Study." *Br J Psychiatry* 193, no. 2 (2008): 108–13.

Lundberg, U. "Stress Hormones in Health and Illness: The Roles of Work and Gender." *Psychoneuroendocrinology* 30, no. 10 (2005): 1017–21.

Nidich, S. I., M. V. Rainforth, D. A. Haaga, J. Hagelin, J. W. Salerno, F. Travis, M. Tanner, C. Gaylord-King, S. Grosswald, and R. H. Schneider. "A Randomized Controlled Trial on Effects of the Transcendental Meditation Program on Blood Pressure, Psychological Distress, and Coping in Young Adults." *Am J Hypertens* 22, no. 12 (2009): 1326–31.

Rainforth, M. V., R. H. Schneider, S. I. Nidich, C. Gaylord-King, J. W. Salerno, and J. W. Anderson. "Stress Reduction Programs in Patients with Elevated Blood Pressure: A Systematic Review and Meta-Analysis." *Curr Hypertens Rep* 9, no. 6 (2007): 520–8.

Salanitro, A. H., E. Funkhouser, B. S. Agee, J. J. Allison, J. H. Halanych, T. K. Houston, M. S. Litaker, D. A. Levine, and M. M. Safford. "Multiple Uncontrolled Conditions and Blood Pressure Medication Intensification: An Observational Study." *Implement Sci* 5 (2010): 55.

"Stress and High Blood Pressure: What's the Connection?" MayoClinic.com., http://www.mayoclinic.com/health/stress-and-high-blood-pressure/hi00092. (Accessed 8/10/10)

Stress can give you a heart attack

Engber, D. "Did Stress Kill Ken Lay?" *Slate* (2006), http://www.slate.com/id/2145074.

Fogoros, R. N. "Does Stress Really Cause Heart Disease?" About.com.

French, D. P., T. M. Marteau, V. Senior, and J. Weinman. "The Structure of Beliefs About the Causes of Heart Attacks: A Network Analysis." *Br J Health Psychol* 7, pt. 4 (2002): 463–79.

Ho, R. C., L. F. Neo, A. N. Chua, A. A. Cheak, and A. Mak. "Research on Psychoneuroimmunology: Does Stress Influence Immunity and Cause Coronary Artery Disease?" *Ann Acad Med Singapore* 39, no. 3 (2010): 191–6.

Ising, H., W. Babisch, and B. Kruppa. "Noise-Induced Endocrine Effects and Cardiovascular Risk." *Noise Health* 1, no. 4 (1999): 37–48.

Lundberg, U. "Stress Hormones in Health and Illness: The Roles of Work and Gender." *Psychoneuroendocrinology* 30, no. 10 (2005): 1017–21.

Martin, B. "Does Stress Cause Heart Disease." PsychCentral, http://psychcentral.com/lib/2006/does-stress-cause-heart-disease/. (Accessed 6/16/10.)

You should stretch before you exercise

Burfoot, A. "Does Stretching Prevent Injuries? Advice from Runner's World." RunnersWorld.com (2010), http://www.runnersworld.com/article/0,7120,s6-241-287-7001-0,00.html. (Accessed 10/7/10.)

"CDC: Stretching Doesn't Prevent Injuries" MSNBC.com. (2010), http://www.msnbc.msn.com/id/4619394/. (Accessed 10/7/10.)

Fradkin, A. J., B. J. Gabbe, and P. A. Cameron. "Does Warming Up Prevent Injury in Sport? The Evidence from Randomised Controlled Trials" *J Sci Med Sport* 9, no. 3 (2006): 214–20.

Hart, L. "Effect of Stretching on Sport Injury Risk: A Review." *Clin J Sport Med* 15, no. 2 (2005): 113.

Herbert, R. D., and M. de Noronha. "Stretching to Prevent or Reduce Muscle Soreness After Exercise." *Cochrane Database Syst Rev* no. 4 (2007): CD004577.

Reynolds, G. "Phys Ed: Does Stretching Before Running Prevent Injuries?" NYTimes.com (2010), http://well.blogs.nytimes.com/2010/09/01/phys-ed-does-stretching-before-running-prevent-injuries/. (Accessed 10/7/10.)

Thacker, S. B., J. Gilchrist, D. F. Stroup, and C. D. Kimsey, Jr. "The Impact of Stretching on Sports Injury Risk: A Systematic Review of the Literature." *Med Sci Sports Exerc* 36, no. 3 (2004): 371–8.

Wingfield, K., G. O. Matheson, and W. H. Meeuwisse. "Preparticipation Evaluation: An Evidence-Based Review." *Clin J Sport Med* 14, no. 3 (2004): 109–22.

Eating sugar causes diabetes

"Can Too Much Sugar Cause Diabetes?" NineMSN.com (2006), http://health.ninemsn.com.au/whatsgoodforyou/theshow/694040/can-too-much-sugar-cause-diabetes.

Curhan, G. C., and J. P. Forman. "Sugar-Sweetened Beverages and Chronic Disease." *Kidney Int* 77, no. 7 (2010): 569–70.

"Diabetes Myths." American Diabetes Association. http://www.diabetes.org/diabetes-basics/diabetes-myths/. (Accessed 6/16/10.)

Malik, V. S., M. B. Schulze, and F. B. Hu. "Intake of Sugar-Sweetened Beverages and Weight Gain: A Systematic Review." *Am J Clin Nutr* 84, no. 2 (2006): 274–88.

Odegaard, A. O., W. P. Koh, K. Arakawa, M. C. Yu, and M. A. Pereira. "Soft Drink and Juice Consumption and Risk of Physician-Diagnosed Incident Type 2 Diabetes: The Singapore Chinese Health Study." *Am J Epidemiol* 171, no. 6 (2010): 701–8.

Rai, M., and J. Kishore. "Myths About Diabetes and Its Treatment in North Indian Population." *Int J Diabetes Dev Ctries* 29, no. 3 (2009): 129–32.

Schulze, M. B., J. E. Manson, D. S. Ludwig, G. A. Colditz, M. J. Stampfer, W. C. Willett, and F. B. Hu. "Sugar-Sweetened Beverages, Weight Gain, and Incidence of Type 2 Diabetes in Young and Middle-Aged Women." *JAMA* 292, no. 8 (2004): 927–34.

Skelly, A. H., M. Dougherty, W. M. Gesler, A. C. Soward, D. Burns, and T. A. Arcury. "African American Beliefs About Diabetes." *West J Nurs Res* 28, no. 1 (2006): 9–29; discussion 30–41.

Sitting too close to the TV will ruin your eyes

"Frequently Asked Questions." University of Michigan Kellogg Eye Center, http://www.kellogg.umich.edu/patientcare/conditions/faq.html#computers. (Accessed 6/30/10.)

O'Connor, A. "The Claim: Sitting Too Close to the TV Is Bad for Your Eyes." *New York Times* (2005), http://www.nytimes.com/2005/06/07/health/07really.html?_r=1.

"Vision Myths." University of Illinois Eye & Ear Infirmary. *The Eye Digest* (2009), http://www.agingeye.net/visionbasics/visionmyths.php.

"You'll Go Blind: Does Watching Television Close-up Really Harm Eyesight?" EarthTalk (2010), http://www.scientificamerican.com/article.cfm?id=earth-talk-tv-eyesight.

Touching a toilet seat will make you sick

Boone, S. A., and C. P. Gerba. "The Occurrence of Influenza A Virus on Household and Day Care Center Fomites." *J Infect* 51, no. 2 (2005): 103–9.

"Fact Sheet: *Trichomonas* Infection." Centers for Disease Control and Prevention, http://www.cdc.gov/ncidod/dpd/parasites/trichomonas/factsht_trichomonas.htm.

Ford, A. "Can Toilet Seats Make You Sick?" DivineCaroline, http://www.divinecaroline.com/22178/77250-toilet-seats-make-sick/3. (Accessed 6/30/10.)

Spencer, D. "6 Items You Touch Every Day That Are Filthier than a Toilet." Cracked.com, http://www.cracked.com/article_17495_6-items-you-touch-every-day-that-are-filthier-than-toilet.html.

"What Can You Catch in Restrooms?" WebMD.com, http://www.webmd.com/balance/features/what-can-you-catch-in-restrooms.

Williams, D. "Is Your Desk Making You Sick?" CNN.com, http://www.cnn.com/2004/HEALTH/12/13/cold.flu.desk/index.html.

You can get gonorrhea from the toilet seat

Allyson, D. "What STDs Can You Get from a Toilet Seat." eHow.com, http://www.ehow.com/facts_5003861_what-stds-can-toilet-seat.html. (Accessed 6/29/10.)

Dayan, L. "Transmission of Neisseria Gonorrhoeae from a Toilet Seat." *Sex Transm Infect* 80, no. 4 (2004): 327.

"Herpes Myths vs. Facts." International Herpes Resource Center, http://www.herpesresourcecenter.com/mvf.html. (Accessed 6/29/10.)

"What Can You Catch in Restrooms?" WebMD, http://www.webmd.com/balance/features/what-can-you-catch-in-restrooms?page=2. (Accessed 6/29/10.)

You shouldn't get a vaccine if you are sick

Brody, J. A., and R. McAlister. "Depression of Tuberculin Sensitivity Following Measles Vaccination." *Am Rev Respir Dis* 90 (1964): 607–11.

Brody, J. A., T. Overfield, and L. M. Hammes. "Depression of the Tuberculin Reaction by Viral Vaccines." *N Engl J Med* 271 (1964): 1294–6.

Ganguly, R., C. L. Cusumano, and R. H. Waldman. "Suppression of Cell-Mediated Immunity After Infection with Attenuated Rubella Virus." *Infect Immun* 13, no. 2 (1976): 464–9.

Hirsch, R. L., F. Mokhtarian, D. E. Griffin, B. R. Brooks, J. Hess, and R. T. Johnson. "Measles Virus Vaccination of Measles Seropositive Individuals Suppresses Lymphocyte Proliferation and Chemotactic Factor Production." *Clin Immunol Immunopathol* 21, no. 3 (1981): 341–50.

Kupers, T. A., J. M. Petrich, A. W. Holloway, and J. W. St Geme, Jr. "Depression of Tuberculin Delayed Hypersensitivity by Live Attenuated Mumps Virus." *J Pediatr* 76, no. 5 (1970): 716–21.

Offit, P. A., J. Quarles, M. A. Gerber, C. J. Hackett, E. K. Marcuse, T. R. Kollman, B. G. Gellin, and S. Landry. "Addressing Parents' Concerns: Do Multiple Vaccines Overwhelm or Weaken the Infant's Immune System?" *Pediatrics* 109, no. 1 (2002): 124–9.

Otto, S., B. Mahner, I. Kadow, J. F. Beck, S. K. Wiersbitzky, and R. Bruns. "General Non-Specific Morbidity Is Reduced After Vaccination within the Third Month of Life—The Greifswald Study." *J Infect* 41, no. 2 (2000): 172–5.

Starr, S., and S. Berkovich. "Effects of Measles, Gamma-Globulin-Modified Measles and Vaccine Measles on the Tuberculin Test." *N Engl J Med* 270 (1964): 386–91.

Zweiman, B., D. Pappagianis, H. Maibach, and E. A. Hildreth. "Effect of Measles Immunization on Tuberculin Hypersensitivity and in Vitro Lymphocyte Reactivity." *Int Arch Allergy Appl Immunol* 40, no. 6 (1971): 834–41.

Getting the flu vaccine is more important for adults than children

Gupta, S. "Health: Flu Shots for Tots." *Time*, 27 October 2003.

Hendrick, B. "Swine Flu Pandemic Hit Children the Hardest." WebMD Health News (2010), http://www.webmd.com/cold-and-flu/news/20100729/swine-flu-pandemic-hit-children-the-hardest.

Lauerman, J. "Flu Shots Halve Risk of Death, Cut Illness in Elderly." Bloomberg.com (2007), http://www.bloomberg.com/apps/news?pid=20601081&sid=aoDQn_PvtPGw&refer=Australia.

Sherman, F. T. "Flu Shots for All Ages." *Geriatrics* 62, no. 11 (2007): 11.

Smith, I. K. "Who Should Get Flu Shots?" *Time* 158, no. 21 (2001): 102.

Too many vaccines will weaken your immune system

Black, R. "Jenny McCarthy and Amanda Peet Duke It Out over Childhood Vaccines and Autism." *New York Daily News* (2008), http://www.nydailynews.com/gossip/2008/09/30/2008-09-30_jenny_mccarthy_and_amanda_peet_duke_it_o.html.

Brunell, P. A., V. M. Novelli, S. V. Lipton, and B. Pollock. "Combined Vaccine Against Measles, Mumps, Rubella, and Varicella." *Pediatrics* 81, no. 6 (1988): 779–84.

Dashefsky, B., E. Wald, N. Guerra, and C. Byers. "Safety, Tolerability, and Immunogenicity of Concurrent Administration of Haemophilus Influenzae Type B Conjugate Vaccine (Meningococcal Protein Conjugate) with Either Measles-

Mumps-Rubella Vaccine or Diphtheria-Tetanus-Pertussis and Oral Poliovirus Vaccines in 14- to 23-Month-Old Infants." *Pediatrics* 85, no. 4, pt. 2 (1990): 682–9.

Davidson, M., G. W. Letson, J. I. Ward, A. Ball, L. Bulkow, P. Christenson, and J. D. Cherry. "DTP Immunization and Susceptibility to Infectious Diseases. Is There a Relationship?" *Am J Dis Child* 145, no. 7 (1991): 750–4.

Deforest, A., S. S. Long, H. W. Lischner, J. A. Girone, J. L. Clark, R. Srinivasan, T. G. Maguire, S. A. Diamond, R. P. Schiller, and E. P. Rothstein et al. "Simultaneous Administration of Measles-Mumps-Rubella Vaccine with Booster Doses of Diphtheria-Tetanus-Pertussis and Poliovirus Vaccines." *Pediatrics* 81, no. 2 (1988): 237–46.

Destefano, F., R. A. Goodman, and G. R. Noble. "Simultaneous Administration of Influenza and Pneumococcal Vaccines." *JAMA* 247 (1992): 2551–54.

Giammanco, G., S. Li Volti, L. Mauro, G. G. Bilancia, I. Salemi, P. Barone, and S. Musumeci. "Immune Response to Simultaneous Administration of a Recombinant DNA Hepatitis B Vaccine and Multiple Compulsory Vaccines in Infancy." *Vaccine* 9, no. 10 (1991): 747–50.

Gregson, A. L., and R. Edelman. "Does Antigenic Overload Exist? The Role of Multiple Immunizations in Infants." *Immunol Allergy Clin North Am* 23, no. 4 (2003): 649–64.

Hilton, S., M. Petticrew, and K. Hunt. "'Combined Vaccines Are like a Sudden Onslaught to the Body's Immune System': Parental Concerns About Vaccine 'Overload' and 'Immune-Vulnerability.'" *Vaccine* 24, no. 20 (2006): 4321–7.

Leask, J., S. Chapman, and S. C. Cooper Robbins. "'All Manner of Ills': The Features of Serious Diseases Attributed to Vaccination." *Vaccine* 28, no. 17 (2010): 3066–70.

Offit, P. A., J. Quarles, M. A. Gerber, C. J. Hackett, E. K. Marcuse, T. R. Kollman, B. G. Gellin, and S. Landry. "Addressing Parents' Concerns: Do Multiple Vaccines Overwhelm or Weaken the Infant's Immune System?" *Pediatrics* 109, no. 1 (2002): 124–9.

Otto, S., B. Mahner, I. Kadow, J. F. Beck, S. K. Wiersbitzky, and R. Bruns. "General Non-Specific Morbidity Is Reduced After Vaccination Within the Third Month of Life—The Greifswald Study." *J Infect* 41, no. 2 (2000): 172–5.

Shinefield, H. R., S. B. Black, B. O. Staehle, T. Adelman, K. Ensor, A. Ngai, C. J. White, S. R. Bird, H. Matthews, and B. J. Kuter. "Safety, Tolerability and Immunogenicity of Concomitant Injections in Separate Locations of M-M-R Ii, Varivax and Tetramune in Healthy Children vs. Concomitant Injections of M-M-R Ii and Tetramune Followed Six Weeks Later by varivax." *Pediatr Infect Dis J* 17, no. 11 (1998): 980–5.

I have just the thing for that cold . . . Vitamin C

Douglas, R. M., H. Hemila, R. D'Souza, E. B. Chalker, and B. Treacy. "Vitamin C for Preventing and Treating the Common Cold." *Cochrane Database Syst Rev* 4 (2004): CD000980.

Gorton, H. C., and K. Jarvis. "The Effectiveness of Vitamin C in Preventing and Relieving the Symptoms of Virus-Induced Respiratory Infections." *J Manipulative Physiol Ther* 22, no. 8 (1999): 530–3.

Masek, J., F. Hruba, M. Neradilova, and S. Hejda. "The Role of Vitamin C in the Treatment of Acute Infections of the Upper Respiratory Pathways." *Acta Vitaminol Enzymol* 28, no. 1–4 (1974): 85–95.

Strohle, A., and A. Hahn. "Vitamin C and Immune Function." *Med Monatsschr Pharm* 32, no. 2 (2009): 49–54; quiz 55–6.

Van Straten, M., and P. Josling. "Preventing the Common Cold with a Vitamin C Supplement: A Double-Blind, Placebo-Controlled Survey." *Adv Ther* 19, no. 3 (2002): 151–9.

Vitamin E helps scars heal

Baumann, L. S., and J. Spencer. "The Effects of Topical Vitamin E on the Cosmetic Appearance of Scars." *Dermatol Surg* 25, no. 4 (1999): 311–5.

Chen, M. A., and T. M. Davidson. "Scar Management: Prevention and Treatment Strategies." *Curr Opin Otolaryngol Head Neck Surg* 13, no. 4 (2005): 242–7.

Curran, J. N., M. Crealey, G. Sadadcharam, G. Fitzpatrick, and M. O'Donnell. "Vitamin E: Patterns of Understanding, Use, and Prescription by Health Professionals and Students at a University Teaching Hospital." *Plast Reconstr Surg* 118, no. 1 (2006): 248–52.

Draelos, Z. D. "The Ability of Onion Extract Gel to Improve the Cosmetic Appearance of Postsurgical Scars." *J Cosmet Dermatol* 7, no. 2 (2008): 101–4.

Khoosal, D., and R. D. Goldman. "Vitamin E for Treating Children's Scars. Does It Help Reduce Scarring?" *Can Fam Physician* 52 (2006): 855–6.

Koc, E., E. Arca, B. Surucu, and Z. Kurumlu. "An Open, Randomized, Controlled, Comparative Study of the Combined Effect of Intralesional Triamcinolone Acetonide and Onion Extract Gel and Intralesional Triamcinolone Acetonide Alone in the Treatment of Hypertrophic Scars and Keloids." *Dermatol Surg* 34, no. 11 (2008): 1507–14.

O'Connor, A. "The Claim: Vitamin E Helps Remove Scars." *New York Times* (2007), http://www.nytimes.com/2007/03/13/health/13real.html?_r=1.

Palmieri, B., G. Gozzi, and G. Palmieri. "Vitamin E Added Silicone Gel Sheets for Treatment of Hypertrophic Scars and Keloids." *Int J Dermatol* 34, no. 7 (1995): 506–9.

Perez, O. A., M. H. Viera, J. K. Patel, S. Konda, S. Amini, R. Huo, D. Zell, S. Tadicherla, and B. Berman. "A Comparative Study Evaluating the Tolerability and Efficacy of Two Topical Therapies for the Treatment of Keloids and Hypertrophic Scars." *J Drugs Dermatol* 9, no. 5 (2010): 514–8.

Zurada, J. M., D. Kriegel, and I. C. Davis. "Topical Treatments for Hypertrophic Scars." *J Am Acad Dermatol* 55, no. 6 (2006): 1024–31.

You will get warts from handling frogs or toads

"Does Touching Toads Gives You Warts?" NineMSN.com http://health.ninemsn.com.au/whatsgoodforyou/theshow/693981/does-touching-toads-gives-you-warts. (Accessed 7/1/10.)

Clark, J. "Do Toads Cause Warts?" HowStuffWorks.com http://animals.howstuffworks.com/amphibians/toads-cause-warts3.htm. (Accessed 7/1/10.)

Krautwurst, T. "Nature Myths, Debunked." Mother Earth News, http://www
.motherearthnews.com/Nature-Community/2006-04-01/Nature-Myths.aspx.
(Accessed 7/1/10.)

Prinalgin. "Warts—Don't Blame Frogs and Toads!" AssociatedContent (2006),
http://www.associatedcontent.com/article/96945/warts_dont_blame_frogs_and_
toads.html?cat=70. (Accessed 7/1/10.)

Going outside with wet hair will make you sick

Douglas, R. G., Jr. "Pathogenesis of Rhinovirus Common Colds in Human
Voluteers." Ann Otol Rhinol Laryngol 79, no. 3 (1970): 563–71.

Eccles, R. "Acute Cooling of the Body Surface and the Common Cold." Rhinology
40, no. 3 (2002): 109–14.

Lee, G. M., J. F. Friedman, D. Ross-Degnan, P. L. Hibberd, and D. A. Goldmann.
"Misconceptions About Colds and Predictors of Health Service Utilization." Pediatrics 111, no. 2 (2003): 231–6.

Mirkin, G. "Catch a Cold." http://www.drmirkin.com/morehealth/9941.html.
(Accessed 6/1/10.)

Zuger, A. " 'You'll Catch Your Death!' an Old Wives' Tale? Well . . ." New York
Times, 4 March 2003.

You should uncover a wound at night to let it air out and heal

Beam, J. W. "Occlusive Dressings and the Healing of Standardized Abrasions."
J Athl Train 43, no. 6 (2008): 600–7.

Benabio, Jeffrey. "Skin Care Myths: Cuts Heal Better When You Let Air at
Them." Dermatology Blog, http://thedermblog.com/2008/05/28/skin-care-myths-
cuts-heal-better-when-you-let-air-at-them/. (Accessed 7/7/10.)

Chvapil, M., H. Holubec, and T. Chvapil. "Inert Wound Dressing Is Not Desir-
able." J Surg Res 51, no. 3 (1991): 245–52.

Field, F. K., and M. D. Kerstein. "Overview of Wound Healing in a Moist Environment." Am J Surg 167, no. 1A (1994): 2S–6S.

"First Aid: Cuts, Scrapes and Stiches." FamilyDoctor.org, http://familydoctor
.org/online/famdocen/home/healthy/firstaid/after-injury/041.html. (Accessed
7/7/10.)

O'Connor, A. "The Claim: Wounds Heal Better When Exposed to Air." New
York Times (2006), http://www.nytimes.com/2006/08/01/health/01real.html.

Vogt, P. M., C. Andree, K. Breuing, P. Y. Liu, J. Slama, G. Helo, and E. Eriksson.
"Dry, Moist, and Wet Skin Wound Repair." Ann Plast Surg 34, no. 5 (1995): 493–9;
discussion 99–500.

Winter, G. D. "Some Factors Affecting Skin and Wound Healing." J Tissue Via-
bility 16, no. 2 (2006): 20–3.

You should lick a wound or put a cut finger in your mouth

Associated Press. "Board Reprimands Oregon Teacher for Licking Students'
Wounds." Seattle Times (2005).

Davies, R. "True or False: Licking a Wound Can Promote Healing." Aurora Health Care, http://www.aurorahealthcare.org/yourhealth/healthgate/getcontent.asp?URLhealthgate=%22157011.html%22. (Accessed 7/8/10.)

Jorge, M.T., and L.A. Ribeiro. "Infections in the Bite Site After Envenoming by Snakes of the *Bothrops* Genus." *Journal of Venomous Animals and Toxins* 3, no. 2 (1997).

"Licking Your Wounds: Scientists Isolate Compound in Human Saliva That Speeds Wound Healing." ScienceDaily.com (2008), http://www.sciencedaily.com/releases/2008/07/080723094841.htm. (Accessed 7/8/10.)

Oudhoff, M. J., J. G. Bolscher, K. Nazmi, H. Kalay, W. van 't Hof, A. V. Amerongen, and E. C. Veerman. "Histatins Are the Major Wound-Closure Stimulating Factors in Human Saliva as Identified in a Cell Culture Assay." *FASEB J* 22, no. 11 (2008): 3805–12.

Shmerling, R. "Licking Your Wounds." Aetna InteliHealth.

Warner, J. "Rare Circumcision Ritual Carries Herpes Risk." WebMD.com, http://www.webmd.com/genital-herpes/guide/20061101/rare-circumcision-ritual-carries-herpes. (Accessed 7/8/10.)

Weil, H.-P., and U. Fischer-Brugge. "Potential Hazard of Wound Licking." *New Engl J. Med* 346, no. 17 (2002).

"Wound-Licking Dangers—Medical News from Around the World." CBSMoneyWatch.com (2002), http://findarticles.com/p/articles/mi_m0876/is_2002_Fall/ai_95147891/.

I have just the thing for that cold . . . Zinc

Alexander, T. H., and T. M. Davidson. "Intranasal Zinc and Anosmia: The Zinc-Induced Anosmia Syndrome." *Laryngoscope* 116, no. 2 (2006): 217–20.

Caruso, T. J., C. G. Prober, and J. M. Gwaltney, Jr. "Treatment of Naturally Acquired Common Colds with Zinc: A Structured Review." *Clin Infect Dis* 45, no. 5 (2007): 569–74.

"Does Zinc Help Fight Colds?" *Mayo Clin Womens Healthsource* 13, no. 12 (2009): 8.

Eby, G. A. "Zinc Lozenges: Cold Cure or Candy? Solution Chemistry Determinations." *Biosci Rep* 24, no. 1 (2004): 23–39.

Eby, G. A., III. "Zinc Lozenges as Cure for the Common Cold—A Review and Hypothesis." *Med Hypotheses* 74, no. 3 (2010): 482–92.

Hulisz, D. "Efficacy of Zinc Against Common Cold Viruses: An Overview." *J Am Pharm Assoc* 44, no. 5 (2004): 594–603.

"Zinc for Colds: Not Much Benefit . . . But There Is a Way to Prevent Flu." *Child Health Alert* 25 (2007): 2–3.

Index

About the Authors

Aaron E. Carroll, MD, MS, is an Associate Professor of Pediatrics and Director of the Center for Health Policy and Professionalism Research at the Indiana University School of Medicine. He has earned a BA in Chemistry from Amherst College, an MD from the University of Pennsylvania School of Medicine, and a master's degree in Health Services from the University of Washington. He loves to read, ski, watch TV, collect comic books, build Legos, play video games, blog, talk on the radio, eat good food, drink good alcohol, and lose to his children at Monopoly. He lives with his wife and three children in Carmel, Indiana.

Rachel C. Vreeman, MD, MS, is an Assistant Professor of Pediatrics in the Children's Health Services Research Group at the Indiana University School of Medicine and Co-Director of Pediatric Research for the Academic Model Providing Access to Healthcare (AMPATH) in Kenya. She has earned a BA in English from Cornell University, an MD from the Michigan State University College of Human Medicine, and a master's degree in Clinical Research from Indiana University. She is a voracious reader who occasionally relinquishes her bookworm ways to explore new cities, play the piano, blog, ride her bicycle, take photographs, and laugh with the people she loves. She divides her time between Indianapolis, Indiana, and Eldoret, Kenya.

Aaron and Rachel are the co-authors of *Don't Swallow Your Gum!: Myths, Half-Truths, and Outright Lies About Your Body and Health.*

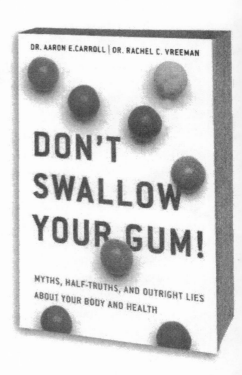